The Anatomy of Stretching

Brad Walker

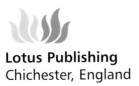

Lotus Publishing
Chichester, England

North Atlantic Books
Berkeley, Californi

D1339107

First published in 2007 by
Lotus Publishing
Apple Tree Cottage, Inlands Road, Nutbourne, PO18 8RJ and
North Atlantic Books
P O Box 12327
Berkeley, California 94712

Drawings Pascale Pollier and Amanda Williams
Text and Cover Design Chris Fulcher
Printed and Bound by Butler Tanner and Dennis Ltd

The Anatomy of Stretching is sponsored by the Society for the Study of Native Arts and Sciences, a nonprofit educational corporation whose goals are to develop an educational and cross-cultural perspective linking various scientific, social, and artistic fields; to nurture a holistic view of arts, sciences, humanities, and healing; and to publish and distribute literature on the relationship of mind, body, and nature.

British Library Cataloguing in Publication Data
A CIP record for this book is available from the British Library
ISBN 978 1 905367 03 0 (Lotus Publishing)
ISBN 978 1 55643 596 6 (North Atlantic Books)

Library of Congress Cataloguing-in-Publication Data

Walker, Brad, 1971-
The anatomy of stretching / Brad Walker.
p. cm.
ISBN-13: 978-1-55643-596-6 (pbk.)
ISBN-10: 1-55643-596-7 (pbk.)
1. Stretching exercises. I. Title.
RA781.63.W35 2006
613.7'182--dc22

2006022377

Contents

How to Use This Book

The Anatomy of Stretching is designed to provide a balance of theoretical information about the fundamentals of stretching and flexibility anatomy and physiology, and the practical application of how to perform 114 unique stretching exercises. All the stretching exercises are indexed according to what part of the body is being stretched and further information is provided on exactly which muscles are being targeted.

As well as a detailed anatomical drawing, each stretch section includes a description of how the stretch is performed, a list of sports and sports injuries that the stretch is most beneficial for, and additional information about any common problems associated with this stretch.

The information about each stretch is presented in a uniform style throughout. An example is given below, with the meaning of headings explained in bold.

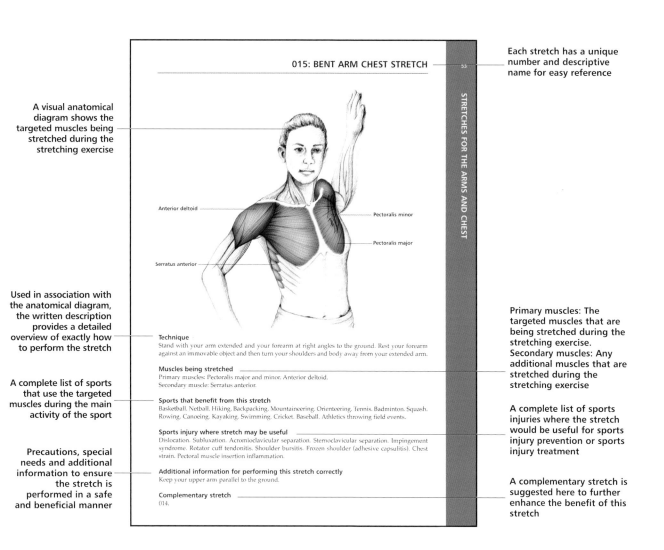

Each stretch has a unique number and descriptive name for easy reference

A visual anatomical diagram shows the targeted muscles being stretched during the stretching exercise

Used in association with the anatomical diagram, the written description provides a detailed overview of exactly how to perform the stretch

A complete list of sports that use the targeted muscles during the main activity of the sport

Precautions, special needs and additional information to ensure the stretch is performed in a safe and beneficial manner

Primary muscles: The targeted muscles that are being stretched during the stretching exercise.
Secondary muscles: Any additional muscles that are stretched during the stretching exercise

A complete list of sports injuries where the stretch would be useful for sports injury prevention or sports injury treatment

A complementary stretch is suggested here to further enhance the benefit of this stretch

015: BENT ARM CHEST STRETCH

STRETCHES FOR THE ARMS AND CHEST

Anterior deltoid

Pectoralis minor

Pectoralis major

Serratus anterior

Technique
Stand with your arm extended and your forearm at right angles to the ground. Rest your forearm against an immovable object and then turn your shoulders and body away from your extended arm.

Muscles being stretched
Primary muscles: Pectoralis major and minor. Anterior deltoid.
Secondary muscle: Serratus anterior.

Sports that benefit from this stretch
Basketball. Netball. Hiking. Backpacking. Mountaineering. Orienteering. Tennis. Badminton. Squash. Rowing. Canoeing. Kayaking. Swimming. Cricket. Baseball. Athletics throwing field events.

Sports injury where stretch may be useful
Dislocation. Subluxation. Acromioclavicular separation. Sternoclavicular separation. Impingement syndrome. Rotator cuff tendonitis. Shoulder bursitis. Frozen shoulder (adhesive capsulitis). Chest strain. Pectoral muscle insertion inflammation.

Additional information for performing this stretch correctly
Keep your upper arm parallel to the ground.

Complementary stretch
014.

Introduction

The subject of stretching and flexibility has evolved considerably over the last ten to fifteen years. Long gone are the days when the topic of stretching was relegated to a few pages at the back of books on health and fitness, or when a dozen stick figures performing the most basic of stretching exercises was considered a detailed reference.

Fifteen years ago it was hard to find a text specifically on stretching, but today there are dozens of references. Everything from "New Age" stretching techniques to martial arts stretching and the very detailed clinical application of stretching for academics has been written.

However, up until now, nothing has covered the topic of the anatomy and physiology behind stretching and flexibility. No book has been able to take you inside the body and show you both the primary and secondary muscles in action during the stretching process. This is where *The Anatomy of Stretching* is different.

The Anatomy of Stretching looks at stretching from every angle, including physiology and flexibility; the benefits of stretching; the different types of stretching; rules for safe stretching; and how to stretch properly. Aimed at fitness enthusiasts of any level, as well as at fitness pros, *The Anatomy of Stretching* also focuses on which stretches are useful for the alleviation or rehabilitation of specific sports injuries.

Written as a visual aid for both athletes and fitness professionals, *The Anatomy of Stretching* gives readers a balance of theoretical information about the fundamentals of stretching and flexibility anatomy and physiology, and the practical application of how to perform 114 unique stretching exercises.

Divided into stand-alone sections, *The Anatomy of Stretching* does not have to be read from cover-to-cover to take advantage of the information it contains. If you want information on stretches for the hamstrings, look under that section; if you want to know how stretching can help you, have a read through some of the benefits in Chapter 2; or if you want to make sure you are stretching properly, refer to the "Rules for Safe Stretching" in Chapter 4.

Whether you are a professional athlete or a fitness enthusiast; a sports coach or personal trainer; a physical therapist or sports doctor, *The Anatomy of Stretching* will benefit you.

1

Physiology and Flexibility

What is Flexibility?

Muscle Anatomy

What is Stretching?

What is Flexibility?

Flexibility is commonly described as the range of movement, or motion, around a particular joint or set of joints. Or in layman's terms, how far we can reach, bend and turn. Tony Gummerson (1990) further expands the general definition by describing flexibility as,

> *"the absolute range of movement in a joint or series of joints that is attainable in a momentary effort with the help of a partner or a piece of equipment."*

Fitness and Flexibility

An individual's physical fitness depends on a vast number of components; flexibility is only one of these. Although flexibility is a vital part of physical fitness it is important to see it as only one spoke in the fitness wheel. Other components include strength, power, speed, endurance, balance, co-ordination, agility and skill.

Although particular sports require different levels of each fitness component it is essential to plan a regular exercise or training program that covers all the components of physical fitness.

Rugby and gridiron for example, rely heavily on strength and power; however the exclusion of skill drills and flexibility training could lead to serious injury and poor performance. Strength and flexibility are of prime concern to a gymnast but a sound training program would also improve power, speed and endurance.

The same is true for each individual: while some people seem to be naturally strong or flexible it would be foolish for such a person to completely ignore the other components of physical fitness. And just because an individual exhibits good flexibility at one joint or muscle group does not mean that the entire individual will be flexible. Therefore flexibility must be viewed as specific to a particular joint or muscle group.

The Dangers and Limitations of Poor Flexibility

Tight, stiff muscles limit our normal range of movement. In some cases, lack of flexibility can be a major contributing factor to muscle and joint pain. In the extreme, lack of flexibility can mean it is difficult, for example, to even bend down or look over our shoulder.

Tight, stiff muscles interfere with proper muscle action. If the muscles cannot contract and relax efficiently, this will result in decreased performance and a lack of muscle movement control. Short, tight muscles also cause a dramatic loss of strength and power during physical activity.

In a very small percentage of cases tight, stiff muscles can even restrict blood circulation. Good blood circulation is vitally important in helping the muscles receive adequate amounts of oxygen and nutrients. Poor circulation can result in increased muscle fatigue and ultimately, the ability to recover from strenuous exercise and the muscles repair process is impeded.

Any one of these factors can greatly increase the chance of becoming injured. Together they present a package that includes muscular discomfort; loss of performance; an increased risk of injury; and a greater likelihood of repeated injury.

How is Flexibility Restricted?

The muscular system needs to be flexible to achieve peak performance and stretching is the most effective way of developing and retaining flexible muscles and tendons. However a number of other factors also contribute to a decrease in flexibility.

Flexibility, or range of movement, can be restricted by both internal and external factors. Internal factors such as bones, ligaments, muscle bulk, muscle length, tendons, and skin all restrict the amount of movement at any particular joint. As an example, the human leg cannot bend forward beyond a straight position because of the structure of the bones and ligaments that make up the knee joint.

External factors such as age, gender, temperature, restrictive clothing and of course any injury or disability will also have an effect on ones flexibility.

Flexibility and the Ageing Process

It is no secret that with each passing year muscles and joints seem to become stiffer and tighter. This is part of the ageing process and is caused by a combination of physical degeneration and inactivity. Although we cannot help getting older, this should not mean that we give up trying to improve our flexibility.

Age should not be a barrier to a fit and active lifestyle but certain precautions should be taken as we get older. Participants just need to work at it for longer, be a little more patient and a lot more careful.

Muscle Anatomy

When aiming to improve flexibility, the muscles and their fascia (sheath) should be the major focus of our flexibility training. While bones, joints, ligaments, tendons, and skin do contribute to our overall flexibility, we have very little control over these factors.

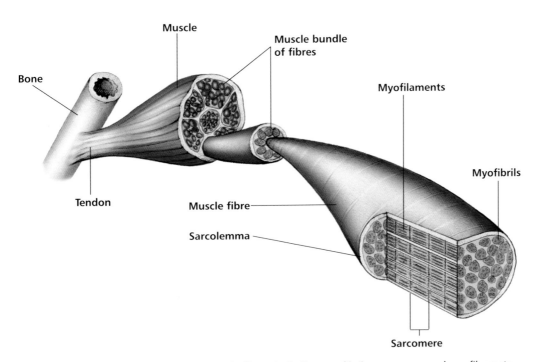

Figure 1.1: A cross-section of muscle fibres, including myofibrils, sarcomeres and myofilaments.

Bones and Joints

Bones and joints are structured in such a way as to allow a specific range of movement. For example, the knee joint will not allow our leg to bend any further forward past a straight leg position, no matter how hard we try.

Ligaments

Ligaments connect bone to bone and act as stabilizers for joints. Stretching the ligaments should be avoided and can result in a permanent reduction of stability at the joint, which can lead to joint weakness and injury.

Tendons

Muscles are connected to the bones by tendons, which consist of dense connective tissue. They are extremely strong yet very pliable. Tendons also play a role in joint stability and contribute less than 10% to a joints overall flexibility, therefore tendons should not be a primary focus of stretching.

Muscles

Muscles are made up of thousands of tiny cylindrical cells called *muscle fibers*. These muscle fibers run parallel to each other and some can be as long as 30 cm.

Within each muscle fiber there are tens of thousands of tiny threads called *myofibrils*. These give the muscle its ability to contract, relax and lengthen. Each myofibril is made up of millions of bands called sarcomeres. Each sarcomere is made up of overlapping thick and thin filaments called *myofilaments*, and each thick and thin myofilament is primarily made up of contractile proteins called *actin* and *myosin*. The muscles and their fascia contain a greater amount of elastic tissue than the other contributing factors mentioned above: therefore these should be the major focus of our flexibility training.

What is Stretching?

Now that we have a general understanding of what flexibility is, let us define stretching. Stretching, as it relates to physical health and fitness, is the process of placing particular parts of the body into a position that will lengthen the muscles and associated soft tissues.

What Happens When a Muscle is Stretched?

Upon undertaking a regular stretching program a number of changes begin to occur within the body and specifically within the muscles themselves. Other tissues that begin to adapt to the stretching process include the ligaments, tendons, fascia, skin and scar tissue.

The process of lengthening the muscles and thereby increasing range of movement begins within the muscles at the sarcomeres. When a particular body part is placed into a position that lengthens the muscle, the overlap between the thick and thin myofilaments begins to decrease. Once this has been achieved and all the sarcomeres are fully stretched, the muscle fiber is at its maximum resting length. At this point further stretching will help to elongate the connective tissues and muscle fascia (sheath). Additionally, G. Goldspink in 1968 and P.E. Williams & G. Goldspink again in 1971 concluded that,

> *"with regular stretching over time, the number of sarcomeres is thought to increase in series, with new sarcomeres added onto the end of existing myofibrils, which in turn, increases the overall muscle length and range of motion."*

2

The Benefits of Stretching

Improved Range of Movement

Increased Power

Reduced Post Exercise Muscle Soreness

Reduced Fatigue

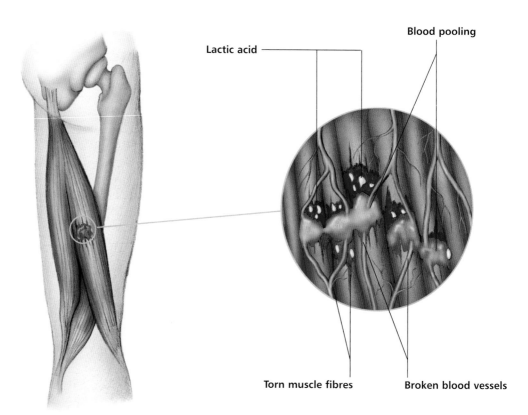

Lactic acid

Blood pooling

Torn muscle fibres

Broken blood vessels

Figure 2.1: Reduced post exercise muscle soreness: micro tears, blood pooling and accumulated waste products.

Stretching is a simple and effective activity that helps to enhance athletic performance, decrease the likelihood of injury and minimize muscle soreness. But how specifically is this accomplished?

Improved Range of Movement

By placing particular parts of the body in certain positions, we are able to increase the length of our muscles. As a result of this, a reduction in general muscle tension is achieved and our normal range of movement is increased.

By increasing our range of movement we are increasing the distance our limbs can move before damage occurs to the muscles and tendons. For example, the muscles and tendons in the back of our legs are put under great strain when kicking a football. Therefore, the more flexible and pliable those muscles are, the further our leg can travel forward before a strain or injury occurs to them.

The benefits of an extended range of movement includes: increased comfort; a greater ability to move freely; and a lessening of our susceptibility to muscle and tendon strain injuries.

Increased Power

There is a dangerous stretching myth that says, "*If you stretch too much you will lose both joint stability and muscle power.*" This is totally untrue. By increasing our muscle length we are increasing the distance over which our muscles are able to contract. This results in a potential increase to our muscles power and therefore increases our athletic ability, while also leading to an improvement in dynamic balance, or the ability to control our muscles.

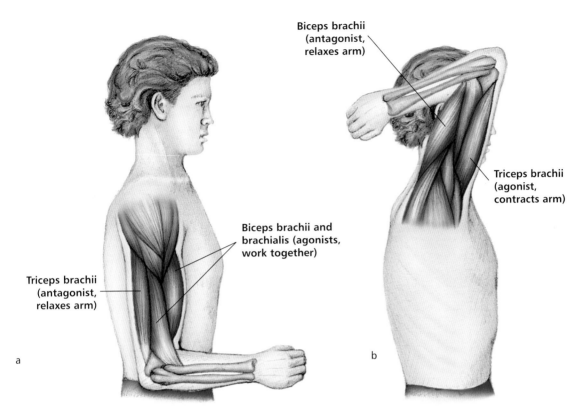

Figure 2.2: a) a tight antagonist causing the agonist to work harder,
b) a normal interaction between agonist and antagonist.

Reduced Post Exercise Muscle Soreness

We have all experienced what happens when we go for a run or to the gym for the first time in a few months. The following day our muscles are tight, sore, stiff and it is usually hard to even walk down a flight of stairs. This soreness that usually accompanies strenuous physical activity is often referred to as *post exercise muscle soreness*. This soreness is the result of micro tears, (minute tears within the muscle fibers), blood pooling and accumulated waste products, such as lactic acid. Stretching, as part of an effective cool-down, helps to alleviate this soreness by lengthening the individual muscle fibers; increasing blood circulation; and removing waste products.

Reduced Fatigue

Fatigue is a major problem for everyone, especially those who exercise. It results in a decrease in both physical and mental performance. Increased flexibility through stretching can help prevent the effects of fatigue by taking pressure off the working muscles, (the agonist). For every muscle in the body there is an opposite or opposing muscle, (the antagonist). If the opposing muscles are more flexible, the working muscles do not have to exert as much force against the opposing muscles. Therefore each movement of the working muscles actually takes less effort.

Added Benefits

Along with the benefits listed above, a regular stretching program will also help to improve posture; develop body awareness; improve co-ordination; promote circulation; increase energy; and improve relaxation and stress relief.

3

Types of Stretching

Static Stretches

    Static Stretching

    Passive Stretching

    Active Stretching

    PNF Stretching

    Isometric Stretching

Dynamic Stretches

    Ballistic Stretching

    Dynamic Stretching

    Active Isolated Stretching

TYPES OF STRETCHING

Stretching is slightly more technical than swinging our leg over a park bench. There are rules and techniques that will maximize the benefits and minimize the risk of injury. In this chapter we will look at the different types of stretching, the particular benefits, risks and uses, plus a description of how each type is performed.

Although there are many different types of stretching, they can all be grouped into one of two categories; static or dynamic.

Static Stretches

The term static stretches refers to stretching exercises that are performed without movement. In other words, the individual gets into the stretch position and holds the stretch for a specific amount of time. Listed below are five different types of static stretching exercises.

Static Stretching

Static stretching is performed by placing the body into a position whereby the muscle (or group of muscles) to be stretched is under tension. Both the antagonist, or opposing muscle group and the agonist, or muscles to be stretched, are relaxed. Then slowly and cautiously the body is moved to increase the tension of the muscle (or group of muscles) to be stretched. At this point the position is held or maintained to allow the muscles to lengthen.

Static stretching is a very safe and effective form of stretching with a limited threat of injury. It is a good choice for beginners and sedentary individuals.

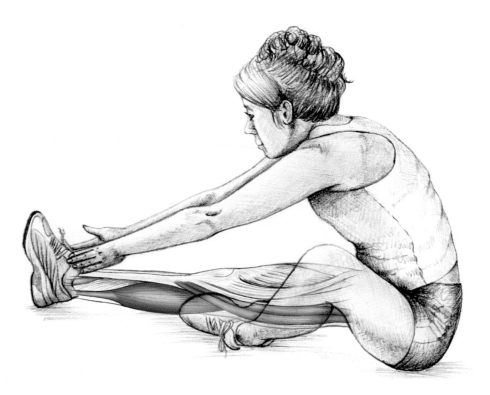

Figure 3.1: An example of static stretching.

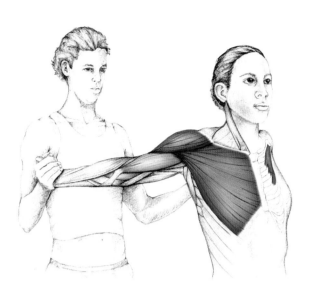

Figure 3.2: An example of passive stretching.

Passive Stretching

This form of stretching is very similar to static stretching; however another person or apparatus is used to help further stretch the muscles. Due to the greater force applied to the muscles, this form of stretching is slightly more hazardous. Therefore it is very important that any apparatus used is both solid and stable. When using a partner it is imperative that no jerky or bouncing force is applied to the stretched muscle. So, choose a partner carefully; the partner is responsible for the safety of the muscles and joints while performing the stretching exercises.

Passive stretching is useful in helping to attain a greater range of movement, but carries with it a slightly higher risk of injury. It can also be used effectively as part of a rehabilitation program or as part of a cool-down.

Active Stretching

Active stretching is performed without any aid or assistance from an external force. This form of stretching involves using only the strength of our opposing muscles (antagonist) to generate a stretch within the targeted muscle group (agonist). The contraction of the opposing muscles helps to relax the stretched muscles. A classic example of an active stretch is one where an individual raises one leg straight out in front as high as possible and then maintains that position without any assistance from a partner or object.

Active stretching is useful as a rehabilitation tool and a very effective form of conditioning before moving onto dynamic stretching exercises. This type of stretching exercise is usually quite difficult to hold and maintain for long periods of time and therefore the stretch position is usually only held for 10–15 seconds.

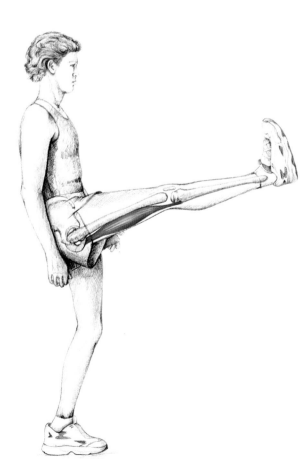

Figure 3.3: An example of active stretching.

PNF Stretching

PNF stretching, or *Proprioceptive Neuromuscular Facilitation*, is a more advanced form of flexibility training that involves both the stretching and contracting of the muscle group being targeted. PNF stretching was originally developed as a form of rehabilitation and for that function it is very effective. It is also excellent for targeting specific muscle groups, and as well as increasing flexibility, (and range of movement) it also improves muscular strength.

The area to be stretched is positioned so that the muscle (or muscle group) is under tension. The individual then contracts the stretched muscle group for 5–6 seconds while a partner applies sufficient resistance to inhibit movement. The effort of contraction should be relevant to the level of conditioning. The contracted muscle group is then relaxed and a controlled stretch is applied for about 30 seconds. The athlete is then allowed 30 seconds to recover and the process is repeated 2–4 times.

Information differs slightly about timing recommendations for PNF stretching. Although there are conflicting responses to the question; *"for how long should I contract the muscle group,"* and *"for how long should I rest between each stretch,"* it is my professional opinion that through a study of research literature and personal experience, the above timing recommendations provide the maximum benefits from PNF stretching.

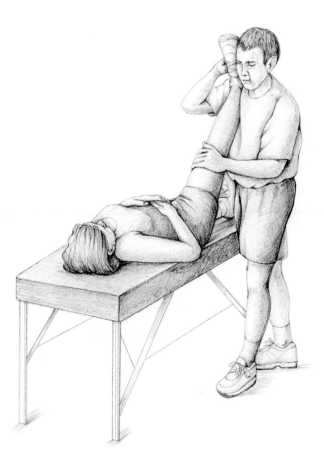

The athlete and partner assume the position for the stretch, and then the partner extends the body limb until the muscle is stretched and tension is felt.

*The athlete then contracts the stretched muscle for 5–6 seconds and the partner must inhibit all movement. The force of the contraction should be relevant to the condition of the muscle. For example, **if the muscle has been injured, do not apply a maximum contraction**.*

The muscle group is relaxed, then immediately and cautiously pushed past its normal range of movement for about 30 seconds. Allow 30 seconds recovery before repeating the procedure 2–4 times.

Figure 3.4: An example of PNF stretching.

Isometric Stretching

Isometric stretching is a form of passive stretching similar to PNF stretching, but the contractions are held for a longer period of time. Isometric stretching places high demands on the stretched muscles and is not recommended for children or adolescents who are still growing. Other recommendations include allowing at least 48 hours rest between isometric stretching sessions and performing only one isometric stretching exercise per muscle group in a session.

A classic example of how isometric stretching is used is the standing 'push-the-wall' calf stretch (*see* Chapter 15, Stretch 097), where the participant stands upright, leans forward towards a wall and then places one foot as far from the wall as is comfortable while making sure that the heel remains on the ground. In this position, the participant would then contract the calf muscles as if trying to push the wall down.

To perform an isometric stretch; assume the position of the passive stretch and then contract the stretched muscle for 10–15 seconds. Be sure that all movement of the limb is restricted. Then relax the muscle for at least 20 seconds. This procedure should be repeated two to five times.

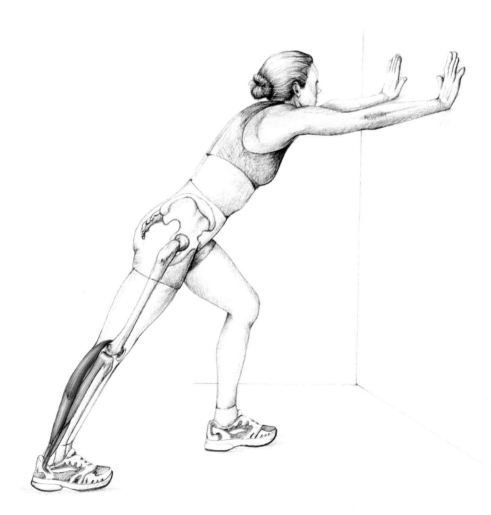

Figure 3.5: An example of isometric stretching.

Dynamic Stretches

The term dynamic stretches refers to stretching exercises that are performed with movement. In other words, the individual uses a swinging or bouncing motion to extend their range of movement and flexibility. Listed below are three different types of dynamic stretching exercises.

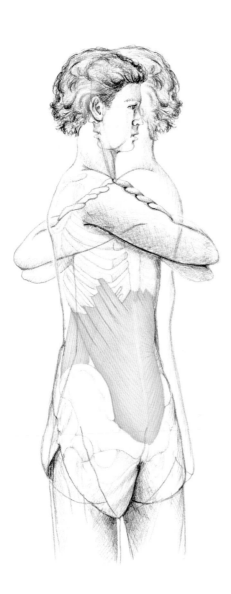

Ballistic Stretching

Ballistic stretching is an outdated form of stretching that uses momentum generated by rapid swinging, bouncing and rebounding movements to force a body part past its usual range of movement.

The risks associated with ballistic stretching far outweigh the gains, especially when better gains can be achieved by using other forms of stretching like dynamic stretching and PNF stretching. Other than potential injury, the main disadvantage of ballistic stretching is that it fails to allow the stretched muscle time to adapt to the stretched position and instead may cause the muscles to tighten up by repeatedly triggering the stretch reflex (discussed in Chapter 4).

Dynamic Stretching

Unlike ballistic stretching (*see* figure 3.3), dynamic stretching uses a controlled, soft bounce or swinging motion to move a particular body part to the limit of its range of movement. The force of the bounce or swing is gradually increased but should never become radical or uncontrolled.

Do not confuse dynamic stretching with ballistic stretching. Dynamic stretching is slow, gentle and very purposeful. At no time during dynamic stretching should a body part be forced past the joints normal range of movement. Ballistic stretching, on the other hand, is much more aggressive and its very purpose is to force the body part beyond the limit of its normal range of movement.

Figure 3.6:
An example of ballistic stretching.

Active Isolated Stretching

Active isolated (AI) stretching is a new form of stretching developed by Aaron L. Mattes. It works by contracting the antagonist, or opposing muscle group, which forces the stretched muscle group to relax. The procedure for performing AI stretching is as follows.

1. Choose the muscle group to be stretched and then get into a position to begin the stretch.
2. Actively contract the antagonist, or opposing muscle group.
3. Move into the stretch quickly and smoothly.
4. Hold for 1–2 seconds and then release the stretch.
5. Repeat five to ten times.

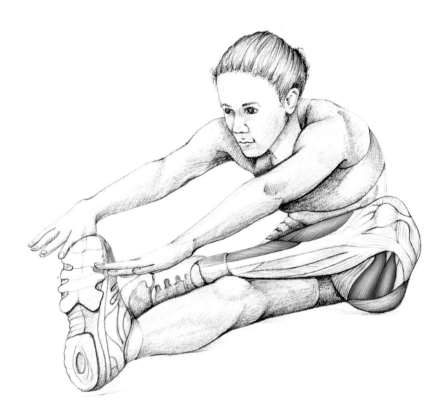

Figure 3.7: An example of active isolated stretching.

4 The Rules for Safe Stretching

Warm-up Prior to Stretching

Stretch Before and After Exercise

Stretch All Major Muscles and Their Opposing
Muscle Groups

Stretch Gently and Slowly

Stretch ONLY to the Point of Tension

Breathe Slowly and Easily While Stretching

As with most activities there are rules and guidelines to ensure that they are safe. Stretching is no exception. Stretching can be extremely dangerous and harmful if done incorrectly. It is vitally important that the following rules be adhered to, both for safety and for maximizing the potential benefits of stretching.

There is often confusion and concerns about which stretches are good and which stretches are bad. In most cases someone has told the inquirer that they should not do this stretch or that stretch, or that this is a good stretch and this is a bad stretch.

Are there only good stretches and bad stretches? Is there no middle ground? And if there are only good and bad stretches, how do we decide which ones are good and which ones are bad? Let us put an end to the confusion once and for all...

There is no such thing as a good or bad stretch!

Just as there are no good or bad exercises, there are no good or bad stretches; only what is appropriate for the specific requirements of the individual. So a stretch that is perfectly okay for one person may not be okay for someone else.

Let me use an example. A person with a shoulder injury would not be expected to do push-ups or freestyle swimming, but that does not mean that these are bad exercises. Now, consider the same scenario from a stretching point of view. That same person should avoid shoulder stretches, but that does not mean that all shoulder stretches are bad.

The stretch itself is neither good nor bad. It is the way the stretch is performed and whom it is being performed on that makes stretching either effective and safe, or ineffective and harmful. To place a particular stretch into a category of "Good" or "Bad" is foolish and dangerous. To label a stretch as "Good" gives people the impression that they can do that stretch whenever and however they want and it will not cause them any problems.

The specific requirements of the individual are what are important!

Remember, stretches are neither good nor bad. However, when choosing a stretch there are a number of precautions and "checks" we need to perform before giving that stretch the okay.

1. Firstly, make a general review of the individual. Are they healthy and physically active, or have they been leading a sedentary lifestyle for the past 5 years? Are they a professional athlete? Are they recovering from a serious injury? Do they have aches, pains or muscle and joint stiffness in any area of their body?

2. Secondly, make a specific review of the area, or muscle group to be stretched. Are the muscles healthy? Is there any damage to the joints, ligaments, tendons, etc.? Has the area been injured recently, or is it still recovering from an injury?

If the muscle group being stretched is not 100% healthy, avoid stretching this area altogether. Work on recovery and rehabilitation before moving onto specific stretching exercises. If however, the individual is healthy and the area to be stretched is free from injury, then apply the following to all stretches.

Warm-up Prior to Stretching

This first rule is often overlooked and can lead to serious injury if not performed effectively. Trying to stretch muscles that have not been warmed is like trying to stretch old, dry rubber bands: they may snap.

Warming-up prior to stretching does a number of beneficial things, but primarily its purpose is to prepare the body and mind for more strenuous activity. One of the ways it achieves this is by helping to increase the body's core temperature while also increasing the body's muscle temperature. By increasing muscle temperature we are helping to make the muscles loose, supple and pliable. This is essential to ensure the maximum benefit is gained from our stretching.

The correct warm-up also has the effect of increasing both our heart rate and respiratory rate. This increases blood flow, which in turn increases the delivery of oxygen and nutrients to the working muscles. All this helps to prepare the muscles for stretching.

A correct warm-up should consist of light physical activity. Both the intensity and duration of the warm-up (or how hard and how long) should be governed by the fitness level of the participating athlete, although a correct warm-up for most people should take about ten minutes and result in a light sweat.

Stretch Before and After Exercise

The question often arises, *"should I stretch before or after exercise?"* This is not an either / or situation; both are essential. It is no good stretching after exercise and counting that as our pre-exercise stretch for next time. Stretching after exercise has a totally different purpose to stretching before exercise. The two are not the same.

The purpose of stretching before exercise is to help prevent injury. Stretching does this by lengthening the muscles and tendons, which in turn increases our range of movement. This ensures that we are able to move freely without restriction or injury occurring.

However, stretching after exercise has a very different role. Its purpose is primarily to aid in the repair and recovery of the muscles and tendons. By lengthening the muscles and tendons, stretching helps to prevent tight muscles and delayed muscle soreness that usually accompanies strenuous exercise.

After exercise our stretching should be done as part of a cool-down. The cool-down will vary depending on the duration and intensity of exercise undertaken, but will usually consist of five to ten minutes of very light physical activity and be followed by five to ten minutes of static stretching exercises.

An effective cool down involving light physical activity and stretching, will help to rid waste products from the muscle, prevent blood pooling, and promote the delivery of oxygen and nutrients to the muscles. All this assists in returning the body to a pre-exercise level, thus aiding the recovery process.

Stretch all Major Muscles and Their Opposing Muscle Groups

When stretching, it is vitally important that we pay attention to all the major muscle groups in the body. Just because a particular sport may place a lot of emphasis on the legs for example, does not mean that one can neglect the muscles of the upper body in a stretching routine.

All the muscles play an important part in any physical activity, not just a select few. Muscles in the upper body for example, are extremely important in any running sport. They play a vital role in the stability and balance of the body during the running motion. Therefore it is important to keep them both flexible and supple.

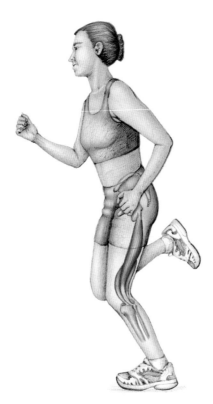

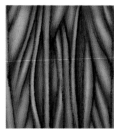

Strained muscle

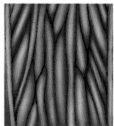

Normal muscle

Figure 4.1: A hamstring tear whilst running, due to tightness of the muscle.

Every muscle in the body has an opposing muscle that acts against it. For example, the muscles in the front of the leg (the quadriceps) are opposed by the muscles in the back of the leg (the hamstrings). These two groups of muscles provide a resistance to each other to balance the body. If one of these groups of muscles becomes stronger or more flexible than the other group, it is likely to lead to imbalances that can result in injury or postural problems.

For example, hamstring tears are a common injury in most running sports. They are often caused by strong quadriceps and weak, inflexible hamstrings. This imbalance puts a great deal of pressure on the hamstrings and can result in a muscle tear or strain.

Stretch Gently and Slowly

Stretching gently and slowly helps to relax our muscles, which in turn makes stretching more pleasurable and beneficial. This will also help to avoid muscle tears and strains that can be caused by rapid, jerky movements.

Stretch ONLY to the Point of Tension

Stretching is NOT an activity that is meant to be painful; it should be pleasurable, relaxing and very beneficial. However many people believe that to get the most from their stretching, they need to be in constant pain. This is one of the greatest mistakes we can make when stretching. Let me explain why.

When the muscles are stretched to the point of pain, the body employs a defense mechanism called the *stretch reflex*. This is the body's safety measure to prevent serious damage occurring to the muscles, tendons and joints. The stretch reflex protects the muscles and tendons by contracting them, thereby preventing them from being stretched.

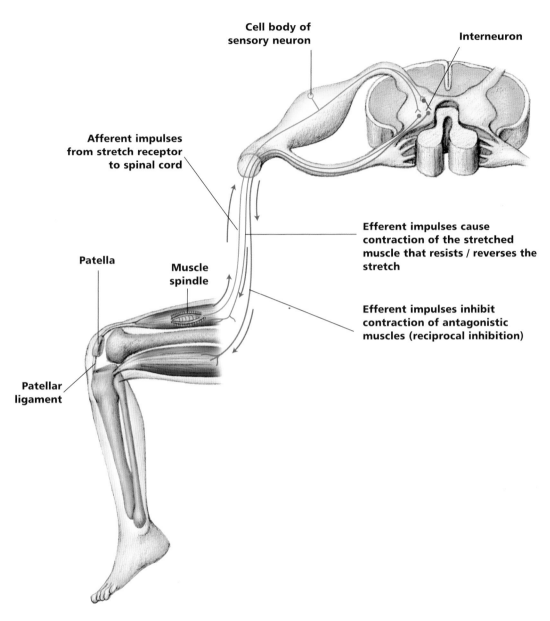

Cell body of sensory neuron

Interneuron

Afferent impulses from stretch receptor to spinal cord

Efferent impulses cause contraction of the stretched muscle that resists / reverses the stretch

Patella

Muscle spindle

Efferent impulses inhibit contraction of antagonistic muscles (reciprocal inhibition)

Patellar ligament

Figure 4.2: The stretch reflex arc.

So to avoid the stretch reflex, avoid pain. Never push the stretch beyond what is comfortable. Only stretch to the point where tension can be felt in the muscles. This way, injury will be avoided and the maximum benefits from stretching will be achieved.

Breathe Slowly and Easily While Stretching

Many people unconsciously hold their breath while stretching. This causes tension in our muscles, which in turn makes it very difficult to stretch. To avoid this, remember to breathe slowly and deeply during all stretching exercises. This helps to relax our muscles, promote blood flow and increase the delivery of oxygen and nutrients to our muscles.

An Example

By taking a look at one of the most controversial stretches ever performed, we can see how the above rules are applied.

The stretch pictured below causes many a person to go into complete meltdown. It has a reputation as a dangerous, bad stretch and should be avoided at all costs.

So why is it that at every Olympic Games, Commonwealth Games and World Championships, sprinters can be seen doing this stretch before their events? Let us apply the above checks to find out.

Firstly, consider the person performing the stretch. Are they healthy, fit and physically active? If not, this is not a stretch they should be doing. Are they elderly, overweight or unfit? Are they young and still growing? Do they lead a sedentary lifestyle? If so, they should avoid this stretch! This first consideration alone would prohibit 50% of the population from doing this stretch.

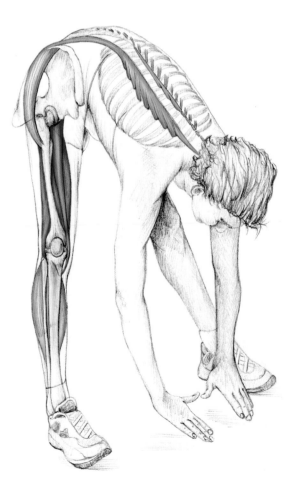

Secondly, review the area to be stretched. This stretch obviously puts a large strain on the muscles of the hamstrings and lower back. So if our hamstrings or lower back are not 100% healthy, do not perform this stretch.

This second consideration would probably rule out another 25%, which means this stretch is only suitable for about 25% of the population: or, the well trained, physically fit, injury free athlete.

Then apply the six precautions above and the well trained, physically fit, injury free athlete can perform this stretch safely and effectively.

Remember, the stretch itself is neither good, nor bad. It is the way the stretch is performed and by whom it is being performed that makes stretching either effective and safe, or ineffective and harmful.

Figure 4.3: Controversial stretch?

5

How to Stretch Properly

When to Stretch

Hold, Count, Repeat

Sequence

Posture

When to Stretch

Stretching needs to be as important as the rest of our training. If we are involved in any competitive type of sport or exercise then it is crucial that we make time for specific stretching workouts. Set time aside to work on particular areas that are tight or stiff. The more involved and committed we are to our exercise and fitness, the more time and effort we will need to commit to stretching.

As discussed earlier it is important to stretch both before and after exercise. But when else should we stretch and what type of stretching is best for a particular purpose?

Choosing the right type of stretching for the right purpose will make a big difference to the effectiveness of our flexibility program. To follow are some suggestions for when to use the different types of stretches.

For warming-up, dynamic stretching is the most effective, while for cooling-down, static, passive and PNF stretching is best. For improving range of movement, try PNF and active isolated stretching, and for rehabilitation, a combination of PNF, isometric and active stretching will give the best results.

So when else should we stretch? Stretch periodically throughout the entire day. It is a great way to keep loose and to help ease the stress of everyday life. One of the most productive ways to utilize our time is to stretch while we are watching television. Start with five minutes of marching or jogging on the spot then take a seat on the floor in front of the television and start stretching.

Competition is a time when great demands are placed on the body; therefore it is vitally important that we are in peak physical condition. Our flexibility should be at its best just before competition. Too many injuries are caused by the sudden exertion that is needed for any sort of competitive sport. Get strict on stretching before competition.

Hold, Count, Repeat

For how long should I hold each stretch? How often should I stretch? For how long should I stretch?

These are the most commonly asked questions when discussing the topic of stretching. Although there are conflicting responses to these questions, it is my professional opinion that through a study of research literature and personal experience, I believe what follows is currently the most correct and beneficial information.

The question that causes the most conflict is: "For how long should I hold each stretch?" Some text will tell us that as little as ten seconds is enough. This is a bare minimum. Ten seconds is only just enough time for the muscles to relax and start to lengthen. For any real benefit to our flexibility we should hold each stretch for at least twenty to thirty seconds.

The time we commit to our stretching will be relative to our level of involvement in our particular sport. So, for people looking to increase their general level of health and fitness, a minimum of about twenty seconds will be enough. However, if we are involved in high-level competitive sport we need to hold each stretch for at least thirty seconds and start to extend that to sixty seconds and beyond.

"How often should I stretch?" This same principle of adjusting our level of commitment to our level of involvement in our sport applies to the number of times we should stretch each muscle group. For example, the beginner should stretch each muscle group two to three times. However, if we are involved at a more advanced level in our sport we should stretch each muscle group three to five times.

"For how long should I stretch?" The same principle applies. For the beginner, about five to ten minutes is enough, and for the professional athlete, anything up to two hours. If we feel that we are somewhere between the beginner and the professional adjust the time we spend stretching accordingly.

Please do not be impatient with stretching. Nobody can get fit in a couple of weeks, so do not expect miracles from a stretching routine. Looking long-term, some muscle groups may need a minimum of three months of intense stretching to see any real improvement. So stick with it, it is well worth the effort.

Sequence

When starting a stretching program it is a good idea to start with a general range of stretches for the entire body, instead of just a select few. The idea of this is to reduce overall muscle tension and to increase the mobility of our joints and limbs.

The next step should be to increase overall flexibility by starting to extend the muscles and tendons beyond their normal range of movement. Following this, work on specific areas that are tight or important for our particular sport. Remember, all this takes time. This sequence of stretches may take up to three months for us to see real improvement, especially if we have no background in agility based activities or are heavily muscled.

No data exists on what order we should do our stretches in. However, it is recommended that we start with sitting stretches, because there is less chance of injury while sitting, before moving on to standing stretches. To make it easier we may want to start with the ankles and move up to the neck or vice-versa. It really does not matter as long as we cover all the major muscle groups and their opposing muscles.

Once we have advanced beyond improving our overall flexibility and are working on improving the range of movement of specific muscles, or muscle groups, it is important to isolate those muscles during our stretching routines. To do this, concentrate on only one muscle group at a time. For example, instead of trying to stretch both hamstrings at the same time, concentrate on only one at a time. Stretching this way will help to reduce the resistance from other supporting muscle groups.

Posture

Posture, or alignment, while stretching is one of the most neglected aspects of flexibility training. It is important to be aware of how crucial it can be to the overall benefits of our stretching. Bad posture and incorrect technique can cause imbalances in the muscles that can lead to injury. While proper posture will ensure that the targeted muscle group receives the best possible stretch.

In many instances a major muscle group can be made up of a number of different muscles. If our posture is sloppy or incorrect, certain stretching exercises may put more emphasis on one particular muscle in that muscle group, thus causing an imbalance that could lead to injury.

For example, when stretching the hamstrings (the muscles at the back of the legs) it is imperative that we keep both feet pointing up. If our feet fall to one side, this will put undue stress on one particular part of the hamstrings, which could result in a muscle imbalance.

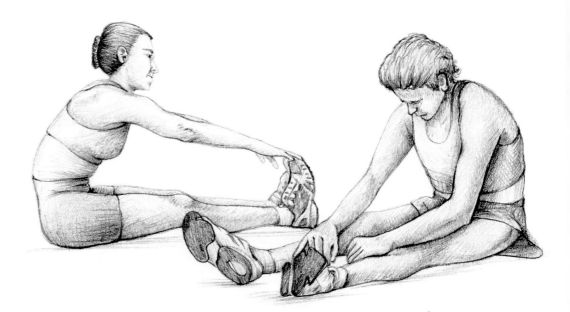

Figure 5.1: The difference between good posture and bad posture.
Note the athlete on the left, feet upright and back relatively straight. The athlete on the right is at greater risk of causing a muscular imbalance that may lead to injury.

6 Stretches for the Neck and Shoulders

001: LATERAL NECK STRETCH

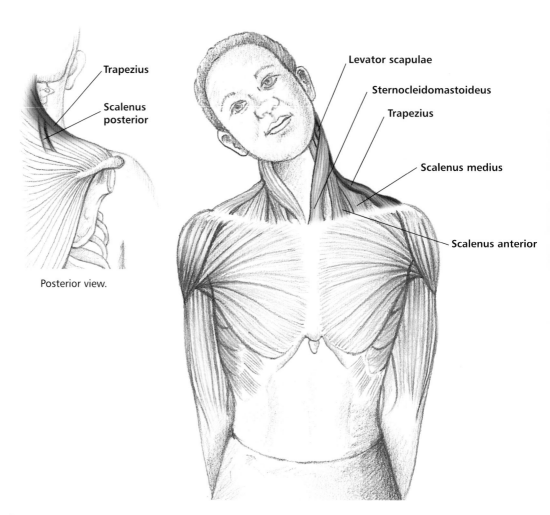

Posterior view.

Technique
Look forward while keeping your head up. Slowly move your ear towards your shoulder while keeping your hands behind your back.

Muscles being stretched
Primary muscles: Levator scapulae. Trapezius.
Secondary muscles: Sternocleidomastoideus. Scalenus anterior, medius and posterior.

Sports that benefit from this stretch
Boxing. American football (gridiron). Rugby. Swimming. Wrestling.

Sports injury where stretch may be useful
Neck muscle strain. Whiplash (neck sprain). Cervical nerve stretch syndrome. Wryneck (acute torticollis).

Additional information for performing this stretch correctly
Keep your shoulders down and your hands behind your back. Do not lift your shoulders up when you tilt your head to the side.

Complementary stretch
002.

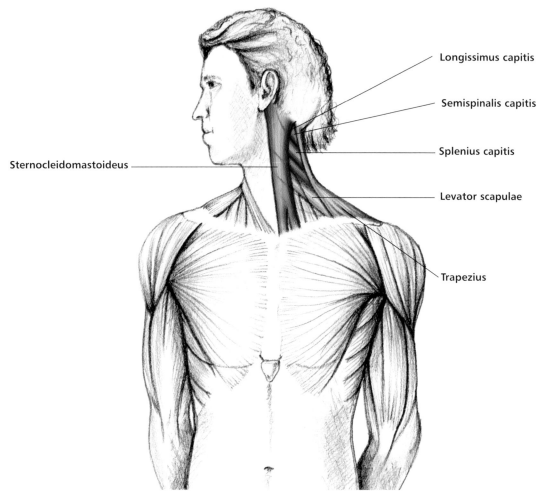

Longissimus capitis

Semispinalis capitis

Splenius capitis

Levator scapulae

Sternocleidomastoideus

Trapezius

Technique
Stand upright while keeping your shoulders still and your head up. Slowly rotate your chin towards your shoulder.

Muscles being stretched
Primary muscles: Sternocleidomastoideus. Splenius capitis. Semispinalis capitis. Longissimus capitis.
Secondary muscles: Levator scapulae. Trapezius.

Sports that benefit from this stretch
Archery. Boxing. American football (gridiron). Rugby. Swimming. Wrestling.

Sports injury where stretch may be useful
Neck muscle strain. Whiplash (neck sprain). Cervical nerve stretch syndrome. Wryneck (acute torticollis).

Additional information for performing this stretch correctly
Keep your head up. Do not let your chin fall towards your shoulders.

Complementary stretch
005.

003: FORWARD FLEXION NECK STRETCH

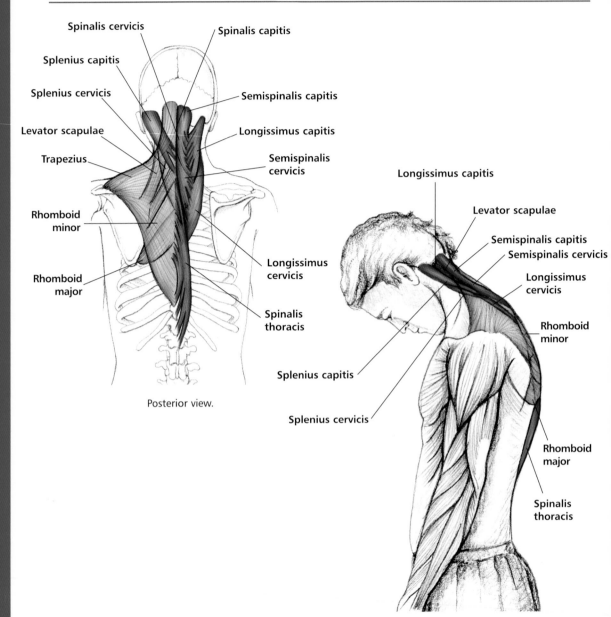

Spinalis cervicis
Splenius capitis
Splenius cervicis
Levator scapulae
Trapezius
Rhomboid minor
Rhomboid major

Spinalis capitis
Semispinalis capitis
Longissimus capitis
Semispinalis cervicis
Longissimus cervicis
Spinalis thoracis

Posterior view.

Longissimus capitis
Levator scapulae
Semispinalis capitis
Semispinalis cervicis
Longissimus cervicis
Rhomboid minor
Splenius capitis
Splenius cervicis
Rhomboid major
Spinalis thoracis

Technique
Stand upright and let your chin fall forward towards your chest. Relax your shoulders and keep your hands by your side.

Muscles being stretched
Primary muscles: Semispinalis capitis and cervicis. Spinalis capitis and cervicis. Longissimus capitis and cervicis. Splenius capitis and cervicis.
Secondary muscles: Levator scapulae. Trapezius. Rhomboids.

Sports that benefit from this stretch
Boxing. American football (gridiron). Rugby. Cycling. Swimming. Wrestling.

Sports injury where stretch may be useful
Neck muscle strain. Whiplash (neck sprain). Cervical nerve stretch syndrome. Wryneck (acute torticollis).

Common problems and additional information for performing this stretch correctly
Some people are more flexible in the upper back and neck than others. Do not over stretch by forcing your head down: instead, relax and let the weight of your head do the stretching for you.

Complementary stretch
006.

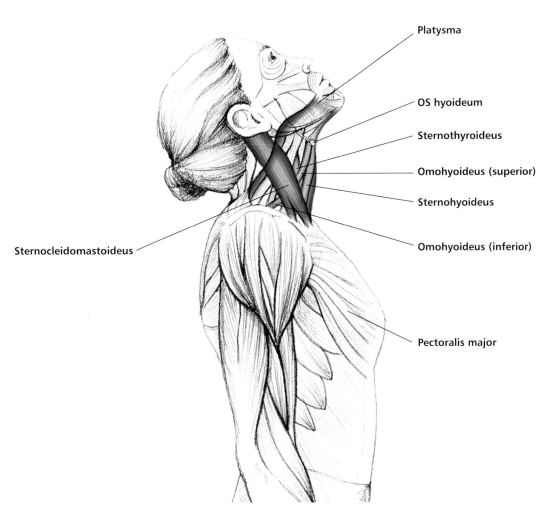

Platysma

OS hyoideum

Sternothyroideus

Omohyoideus (superior)

Sternohyoideus

Omohyoideus (inferior)

Sternocleidomastoideus

Pectoralis major

Technique
Stand upright and lift your head, looking upwards as if trying to point up with your chin. Relax your shoulders and keep your hands by your side.

Muscles being stretched
Primary muscles: Platysma. Sternocleidomastoideus.
Secondary muscles: Omohyoideus. Sternohyoideus. Sternothyroideus.

Sports that benefit from this stretch
Boxing. American football (gridiron). Rugby. Cycling. Swimming. Wrestling.

Sports injury where stretch may be useful
Neck muscle strain. Whiplash (neck sprain). Cervical nerve stretch syndrome. Wryneck (acute torticollis).

Additional information for performing this stretch correctly
Keep your mouth closed and your teeth together when doing this stretch.

Complementary stretch
029.

005: NECK PROTRACTION STRETCH

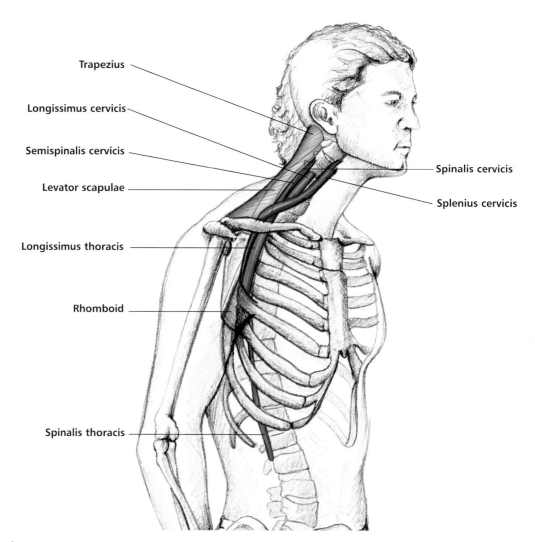

Trapezius

Longissimus cervicis

Semispinalis cervicis

Levator scapulae

Longissimus thoracis

Rhomboid

Spinalis thoracis

Spinalis cervicis

Splenius cervicis

Technique
Keep your head up then push your head forward by sticking your chin out.

Muscles being stretched
Primary muscles: Semispinalis cervicis. Spinalis cervicis. Longissimus cervicis. Splenius cervicis. Secondary muscles: Levator scapulae. Trapezius. Rhomboids.

Sports that benefit from this stretch
Boxing. American football (gridiron). Rugby. Cycling. Swimming. Wrestling.

Sports injury where stretch may be useful
Neck muscle strain. Whiplash (neck sprain). Cervical nerve stretch syndrome. Wryneck (acute torticollis).

Additional information for performing this stretch correctly
Keep your head up. Do not let your chin fall towards the ground.

Complementary stretch
003.

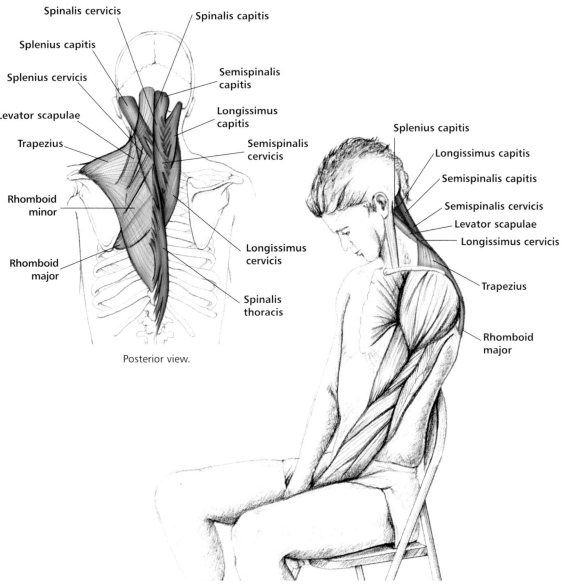

Spinalis cervicis
Spinalis capitis
Splenius capitis
Semispinalis capitis
Splenius cervicis
Longissimus capitis
Levator scapulae
Semispinalis cervicis
Trapezius
Rhomboid minor
Longissimus cervicis
Rhomboid major
Spinalis thoracis

Posterior view.

Splenius capitis
Longissimus capitis
Semispinalis capitis
Semispinalis cervicis
Levator scapulae
Longissimus cervicis
Trapezius
Rhomboid major

Technique
While sitting on a chair, cross your arms over and hang on to the chair between your legs. Let your head fall forward and then lean backwards.

Muscles being stretched
Primary muscles: Semispinalis capitis and cervicis. Spinalis capitis and cervicis. Longissimus capitis and cervicis. Splenius capitis and cervicis.
Secondary muscles: Levator scapulae. Trapezius. Rhomboids.

Sports that benefit from this stretch
Archery. Boxing. American football (gridiron). Rugby. Cycling. Golf. Swimming. Wrestling.

Sports injury where stretch may be useful
Neck muscle strain. Whiplash (neck sprain). Cervical nerve stretch syndrome. Wryneck (acute torticollis).

Common problems and additional information for performing this stretch correctly
Some people are more flexible in the upper back and neck than others. Do not over stretch by forcing your head down: instead, relax and let the weight of your head do the stretching for you.

Complementary stretches
003, 010.

007: PARALLEL ARM SHOULDER STRETCH

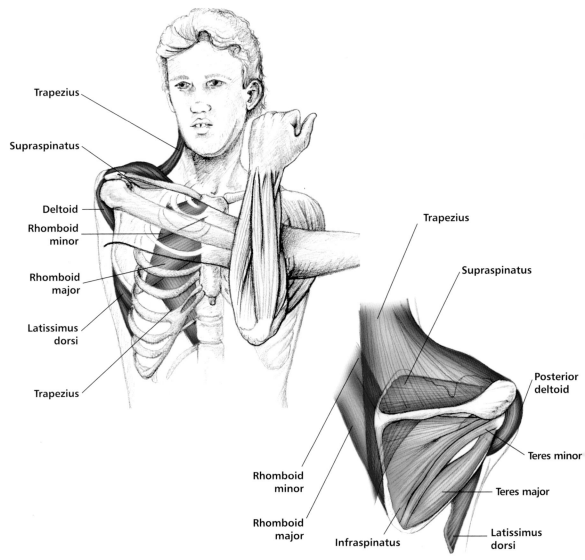

Posterior view.

Technique
Stand upright and place one arm across your body. Keep your arm parallel to the ground and pull your elbow towards your opposite shoulder.

Muscles being stretched
Primary muscles: Trapezius. Rhomboids. Latissimus dorsi. Posterior deltoid.
Secondary muscles: Supraspinatus. Infraspinatus. Teres major and minor.

Sports that benefit from this stretch
Archery. Cricket. Baseball. Softball. Boxing. Golf. Tennis. Badminton. Squash. Rowing. Canoeing. Kayaking. Swimming. Athletics throwing field events.

Sports injury where stretch may be useful
Dislocation. Subluxation. Acromioclavicular separation. Sternoclavicular separation. Impingement syndrome. Rotator cuff tendonitis. Shoulder bursitis. Frozen shoulder (adhesive capsulitis).

Additional information for performing this stretch correctly
Keep your arm straight and parallel to the ground.

Complementary stretch
008.

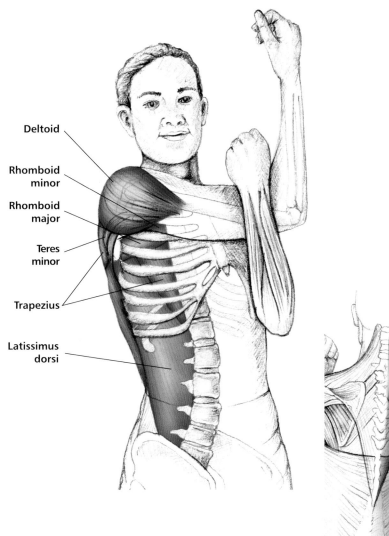

Deltoid

Rhomboid minor

Rhomboid major

Teres minor

Trapezius

Latissimus dorsi

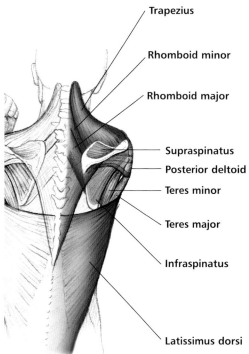

Trapezius

Rhomboid minor

Rhomboid major

Supraspinatus

Posterior deltoid

Teres minor

Teres major

Infraspinatus

Latissimus dorsi

Posterior view.

Technique
Stand upright and place one arm across your body. Bend your arm at 90 degrees and pull your elbow towards your opposite shoulder.

Muscles being stretched
Primary muscles: Trapezius. Rhomboids. Latissimus dorsi. Posterior deltoid.
Secondary muscles: Supraspinatus. Infraspinatus. Teres major and minor.

Sports that benefit from this stretch
Archery. Cricket. Baseball. Softball. Boxing. Golf. Tennis. Badminton. Squash. Rowing. Canoeing. Kayaking. Swimming. Athletics throwing field events.

Sports injury where stretch may be useful
Dislocation. Subluxation. Acromioclavicular separation. Sternoclavicular separation. Impingement syndrome. Rotator cuff tendonitis. Shoulder bursitis. Frozen shoulder (adhesive capsulitis).

Additional information for performing this stretch correctly
Keep your upper arm parallel to the ground.

Complementary stretch
007.

009: WRAP AROUND SHOULDER STRETCH

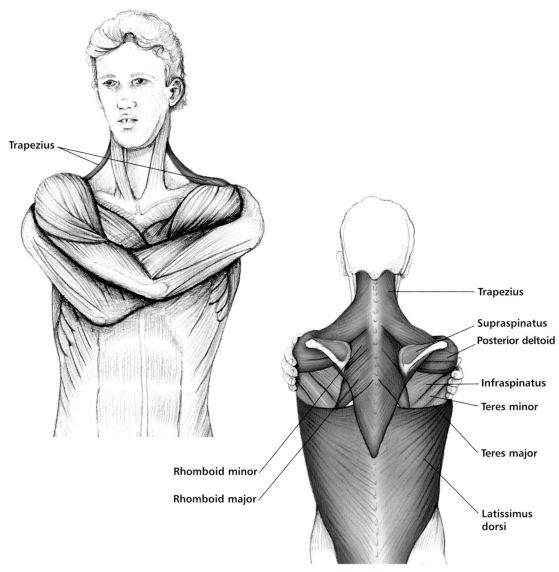

Trapezius

Trapezius

Supraspinatus

Posterior deltoid

Infraspinatus

Teres minor

Teres major

Rhomboid minor

Rhomboid major

Latissimus dorsi

Posterior view.

Technique
Stand upright and wrap your arms around your shoulders as if hugging yourself. Pull your shoulders back.

Muscles being stretched
Primary muscles: Trapezius. Rhomboids. Latissimus dorsi. Posterior deltoid.
Secondary muscles: Supraspinatus. Infraspinatus. Teres major and minor.

Sports that benefit from this stretch
Archery. Cricket. Baseball. Softball. Boxing. Golf. Tennis. Badminton. Squash. Rowing. Canoeing. Kayaking. Swimming. Athletics throwing field events.

Sports injury where stretch may be useful
Dislocation. Subluxation. Acromioclavicular separation. Sternoclavicular separation. Impingement syndrome. Rotator cuff tendonitis. Shoulder bursitis. Frozen shoulder (adhesive capsulitis).

Common problems and additional information for performing this stretch correctly
Do not pull too quickly on your shoulders. Ease into the stretch by slowly pulling your shoulders back.

Complementary stretch
010.

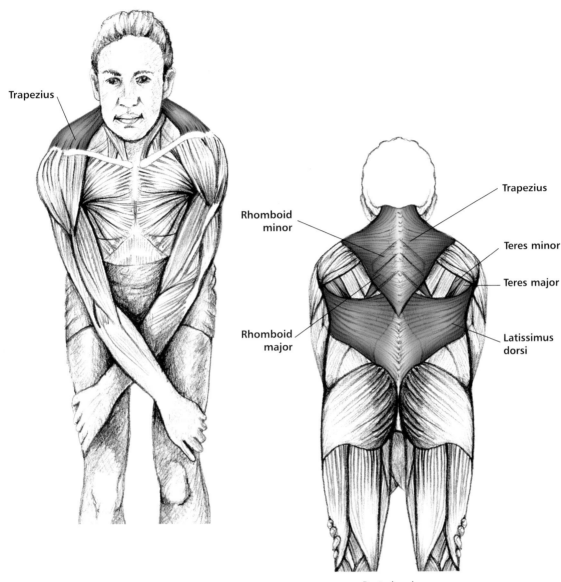

Posterior view.

Technique
Stand with your knees bent. Cross your arms over and grab the back of your knees. Then start to rise upwards until you feel tension in your upper back and shoulders.

Muscles being stretched
Primary muscles: Trapezius. Rhomboids. Latissimus dorsi.
Secondary muscles: Teres major and minor.

Sports that benefit from this stretch
Archery. Cricket. Baseball. Softball. Boxing. Golf. Tennis. Badminton. Squash. Rowing. Canoeing. Kayaking. Swimming. Athletics throwing field events.

Sports injury where stretch may be useful
Dislocation. Subluxation. Acromioclavicular separation. Sternoclavicular separation. Impingement syndrome. Rotator cuff tendonitis. Shoulder bursitis. Frozen shoulder (adhesive capsulitis).

Common problems and additional information for performing this stretch correctly
Keep your shoulders level to the ground and avoid twisting or turning to one side.

Complementary stretch
006.

011: REVERSE SHOULDER STRETCH

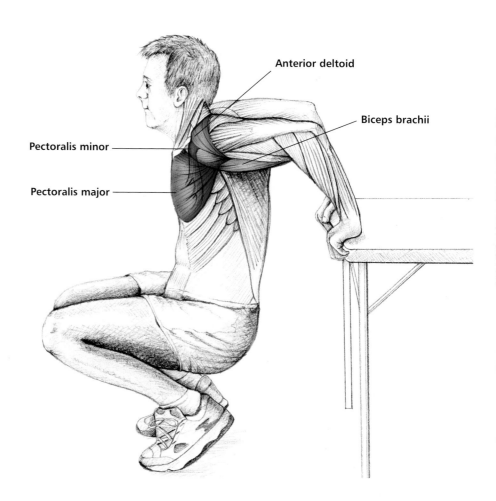

Anterior deltoid

Biceps brachii

Pectoralis minor

Pectoralis major

Technique
Stand upright with your back towards a table or bench and place your hands on the edge of the table or bench. Slowly lower your entire body.

Muscles being stretched
Primary muscles: Anterior deltoid. Pectoralis major and minor.
Secondary muscle: Biceps brachii.

Sports that benefit from this stretch
Archery. Cricket. Baseball. Softball. Boxing. Golf. Tennis. Badminton. Squash. Rowing. Canoeing. Kayaking. Swimming. Athletics throwing field events.

Sports injury where stretch may be useful
Dislocation. Subluxation. Acromioclavicular separation. Sternoclavicular separation. Impingement syndrome. Rotator cuff tendonitis. Shoulder bursitis. Frozen shoulder (adhesive capsulitis). Biceps tendon rupture. Bicepital tendonitis. Biceps strain. Chest strain. Pectoral muscle insertion inflammation.

Common problems and additional information for performing this stretch correctly
Use your legs to control the lowering of your body. Do not lower your body too quickly.

Complementary stretch
016.

7

Stretches for the Arms and Chest

012: ABOVE HEAD CHEST STRETCH

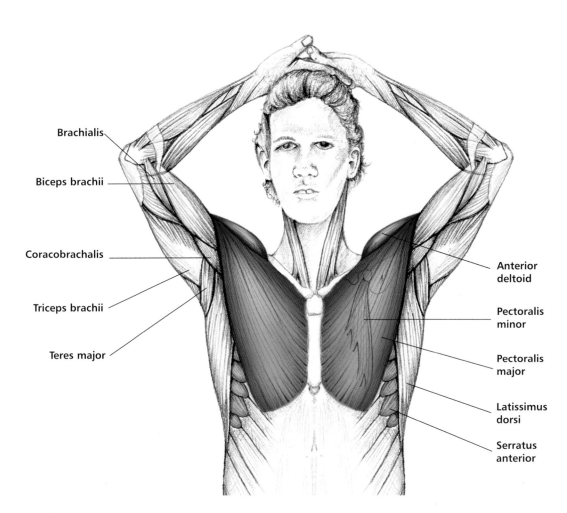

Brachialis

Biceps brachii

Coracobrachialis

Triceps brachii

Teres major

Anterior deltoid

Pectoralis minor

Pectoralis major

Latissimus dorsi

Serratus anterior

Technique
Stand upright and interlock your fingers. Bend your arms and place them above your head while forcing your elbows and hands backwards.

Muscles being stretched
Primary muscles: Pectoralis major and minor. Anterior deltoid.
Secondary muscle: Serratus anterior.

Sports that benefit from this stretch
Basketball. Netball. Hiking. Backpacking. Mountaineering. Orienteering. Tennis. Badminton. Squash. Rowing. Canoeing. Kayaking. Swimming. Cricket. Baseball. Athletics throwing field events.

Sports injury where stretch may be useful
Impingement syndrome. Rotator cuff tendonitis. Shoulder bursitis. Frozen shoulder (adhesive capsulitis). Chest strain. Pectoral muscle insertion inflammation.

Additional information for performing this stretch correctly
Vary the height of your hands. Lower your hands behind your head to place an emphasis on the *anterior deltoid* and raise your hands above your head to emphasize the *pectoral* muscles.

Complementary stretch
017.

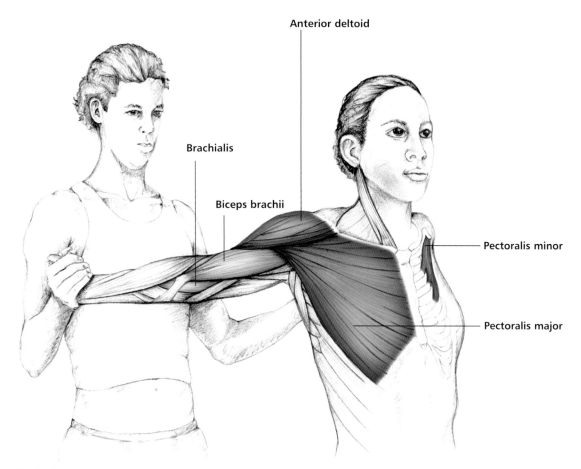

Anterior deltoid

Brachialis

Biceps brachii

Pectoralis minor

Pectoralis major

Technique
Extend both of your arms parallel to the ground. Have a partner hold on to your hands and slowly pull your arms backwards.

Muscles being stretched
Primary muscles: Pectoralis major and minor. Anterior deltoid.
Secondary muscles: Biceps brachii. Brachialis.

Sports that benefit from this stretch
Basketball. Netball. Hiking. Backpacking. Mountaineering. Orienteering. Tennis. Badminton. Squash. Rowing. Canoeing. Kayaking. Swimming. Cricket. Baseball. Athletics throwing field events.

Sports injury where stretch may be useful
Dislocation. Subluxation. Acromioclavicular separation. Sternoclavicular separation. Impingement syndrome. Rotator cuff tendonitis. Shoulder bursitis. Frozen shoulder (adhesive capsulitis). Biceps tendon rupture. Bicepital tendonitis. Biceps strain. Chest strain. Pectoral muscle insertion inflammation.

Additional information for performing this stretch correctly
Keep your arms parallel to the ground and your palms facing outward.

Complementary stretch
014.

014: PARALLEL ARM CHEST STRETCH

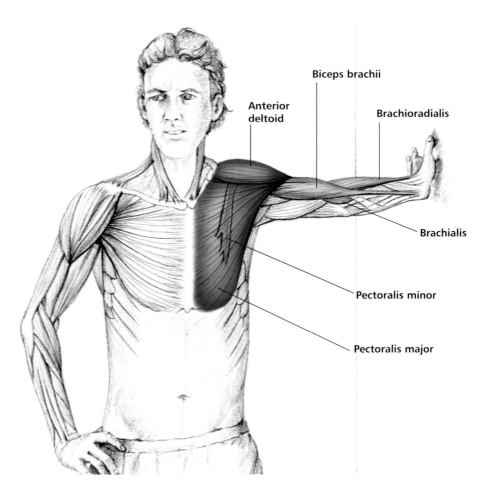

Technique
Stand with your arm extended to the rear and parallel to the ground. Hold on to an immovable object and then turn your shoulders and body away from your outstretched arm.

Muscles being stretched
Primary muscles: Pectoralis major and minor. Anterior deltoid.
Secondary muscles: Biceps brachii. Brachialis. Brachioradialis.

Sports that benefit from this stretch
Basketball. Netball. Hiking. Backpacking. Mountaineering. Orienteering. Tennis. Badminton. Squash. Rowing. Canoeing. Kayaking. Swimming. Cricket. Baseball. Athletics throwing field events.

Sports injury where stretch may be useful
Dislocation. Subluxation. Acromioclavicular separation. Sternoclavicular separation. Impingement syndrome. Rotator cuff tendonitis. Shoulder bursitis. Frozen shoulder (adhesive capsulitis). Biceps tendon rupture. Bicepital tendonitis. Biceps strain. Chest strain. Pectoral muscle insertion inflammation.

Additional information for performing this stretch correctly
Keep your arm parallel to the ground and your fingers pointing backwards.

Complementary stretch
013.

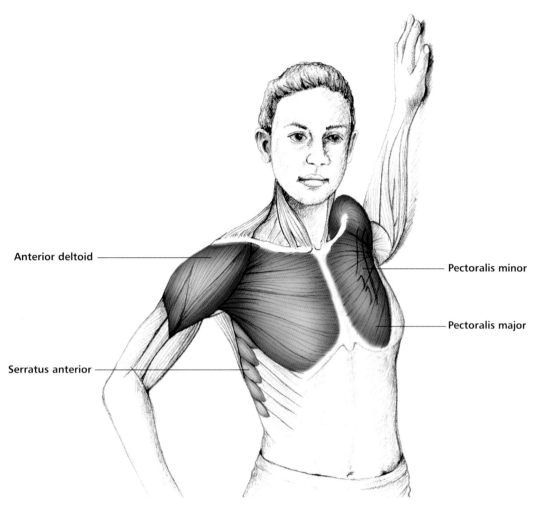

Anterior deltoid

Serratus anterior

Pectoralis minor

Pectoralis major

Technique
Stand with your arm extended and your forearm at right angles to the ground. Rest your forearm against an immovable object and then turn your shoulders and body away from your extended arm.

Muscles being stretched
Primary muscles: Pectoralis major and minor. Anterior deltoid.
Secondary muscle: Serratus anterior.

Sports that benefit from this stretch
Basketball. Netball. Hiking. Backpacking. Mountaineering. Orienteering. Tennis. Badminton. Squash. Rowing. Canoeing. Kayaking. Swimming. Cricket. Baseball. Athletics throwing field events.

Sports injury where stretch may be useful
Dislocation. Subluxation. Acromioclavicular separation. Sternoclavicular separation. Impingement syndrome. Rotator cuff tendonitis. Shoulder bursitis. Frozen shoulder (adhesive capsulitis). Chest strain. Pectoral muscle insertion inflammation.

Additional information for performing this stretch correctly
Keep your upper arm parallel to the ground.

Complementary stretch
014.

016: BEHIND THE BACK CHEST STRETCH

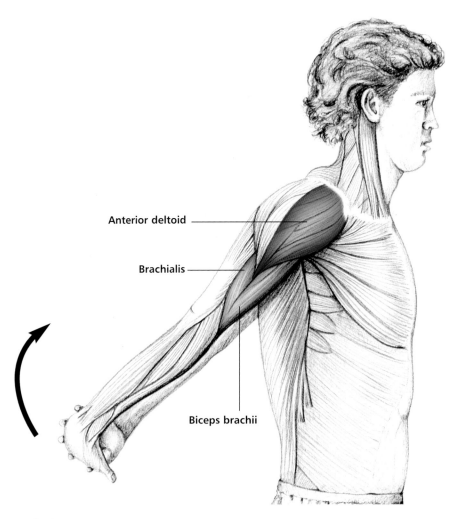

Anterior deltoid

Brachialis

Biceps brachii

Technique
Stand upright and clasp your hands together behind your back. Slowly lift your hands upward.

Muscles being stretched
Primary muscle: Anterior deltoid.
Secondary muscles. Biceps brachii. Brachialis.

Sports that benefit from this stretch
Basketball. Netball. Hiking. Backpacking. Mountaineering. Orienteering. Tennis. Badminton. Squash. Rowing. Canoeing. Kayaking. Swimming. Cricket. Baseball. Athletics throwing field events.

Sports injury where stretch may be useful
Dislocation. Subluxation. Acromioclavicular separation. Sternoclavicular separation. Impingement syndrome. Rotator cuff tendonitis. Shoulder bursitis. Frozen shoulder (adhesive capsulitis). Chest strain. Pectoral muscle insertion inflammation.

Additional information for performing this stretch correctly
Do not lean forward while lifting your hands upward.

Complementary stretch
011.

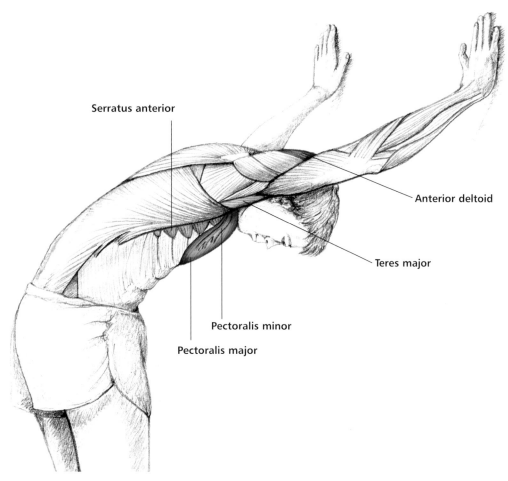

Serratus anterior

Anterior deltoid

Teres major

Pectoralis minor

Pectoralis major

Technique
Face a wall and place both hands on the wall just above your head. Slowly lower your shoulders as if moving your chin towards the ground.

Muscles being stretched
Primary muscles: Pectoralis major and minor. Anterior deltoid.
Secondary muscles: Serratus anterior. Teres major.

Sports that benefit from this stretch
Basketball. Netball. Hiking. Backpacking. Mountaineering. Orienteering. Tennis. Badminton. Squash. Rowing. Canoeing. Kayaking. Swimming. Cricket. Baseball. Athletics throwing field events.

Sports injury where stretch may be useful
Dislocation. Subluxation. Acromioclavicular separation. Sternoclavicular separation. Impingement syndrome. Rotator cuff tendonitis. Shoulder bursitis. Frozen shoulder (adhesive capsulitis). Chest strain. Pectoral muscle insertion inflammation.

Additional information for performing this stretch correctly
Keep your arms straight and your fingers pointing straight upwards.

Complementary stretch
012.

018: TRICEPS STRETCH

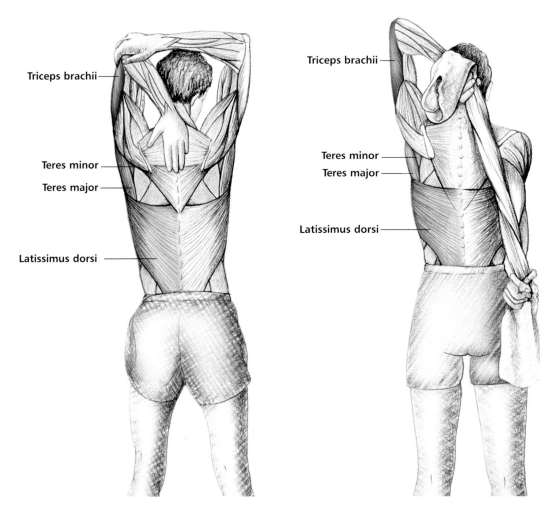

Technique
Stand with your hand behind your neck and your elbow pointing upwards. Then use your other hand (or a rope or towel) to pull your elbow down.

Muscles being stretched
Primary muscle: Triceps brachii.
Secondary muscles: Latissimus dorsi. Teres major and minor.

Sports that benefit from this stretch
Basketball. Netball. Tennis. Badminton. Squash. Rowing. Canoeing. Kayaking. Swimming. Cricket. Baseball. Athletics throwing field events. Volleyball.

Sports injury where stretch may be useful
Elbow sprain. Elbow dislocation. Elbow bursitis. Triceps tendon rupture.

Common problems and additional information for performing this stretch correctly
Do not perform this stretch for an extended period of time, as the blood circulation is restricted in the shoulder.

Complementary stretch
034.

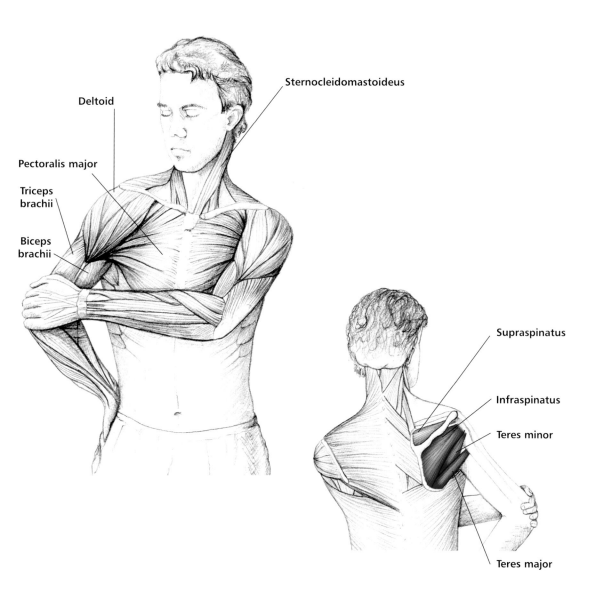

Deltoid

Sternocleidomastoideus

Pectoralis major

Triceps brachii

Biceps brachii

Supraspinatus

Infraspinatus

Teres minor

Teres major

Technique
Stand with your hand behind the middle of your back and your elbow pointing out. Reach over with your other hand and gently pull your elbow forward.

Muscles being stretched
Primary muscles: Infraspinatus. Teres major and minor.
Secondary muscle: Supraspinatus.

Sports that benefit from this stretch
Martial arts. Tennis. Badminton. Squash. Rowing. Canoeing. Kayaking. Swimming. Cricket. Baseball. Athletics throwing field events. Wrestling.

Sports injury where stretch may be useful
Dislocation. Subluxation. Acromioclavicular separation. Sternoclavicular separation. Impingement syndrome. Rotator cuff tendonitis. Shoulder bursitis. Frozen shoulder (adhesive capsulitis).

Common problems and additional information for performing this stretch correctly
Many people are very tight in the rotator cuff muscles of the shoulder. Perform this stretch very slowly to start with and use extreme caution at all times.

Complementary stretch
021.

020: ARM-UP ROTATOR STRETCH

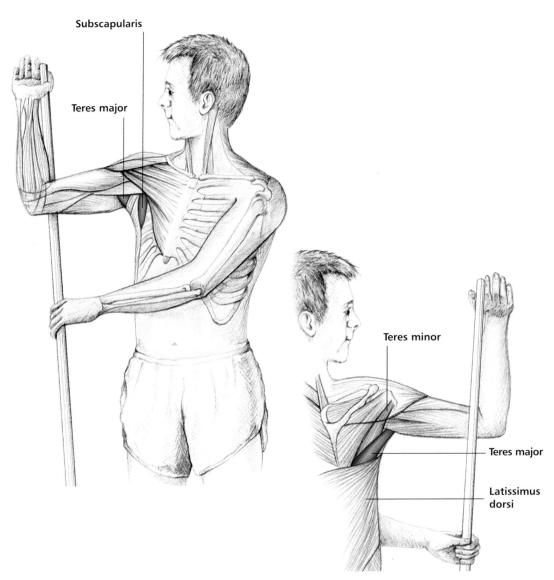

Subscapularis

Teres major

Teres minor

Teres major

Latissimus dorsi

Technique
Stand with your arm out and your forearm pointing upwards at 90 degrees. Place a broomstick in your hand and behind your elbow. With your other hand pull the bottom of the broomstick forward.

Muscles being stretched
Primary muscles: Subscapularis. Teres major. Secondary muscle: Teres minor.

Sports that benefit from this stretch
Martial arts. Tennis. Badminton. Squash. Rowing. Canoeing. Kayaking. Swimming. Cricket. Baseball. Athletics throwing field events. Wrestling.

Sports injury where stretch may be useful
Dislocation. Subluxation. Acromioclavicular separation. Sternoclavicular separation. Impingement syndrome. Rotator cuff tendonitis. Shoulder bursitis. Frozen shoulder (adhesive capsulitis).

Common problems and additional information for performing this stretch correctly
Many people are very tight in the rotator cuff muscles of the shoulder. Perform this stretch very slowly to start with and use extreme caution at all times.

Complementary stretch
021.

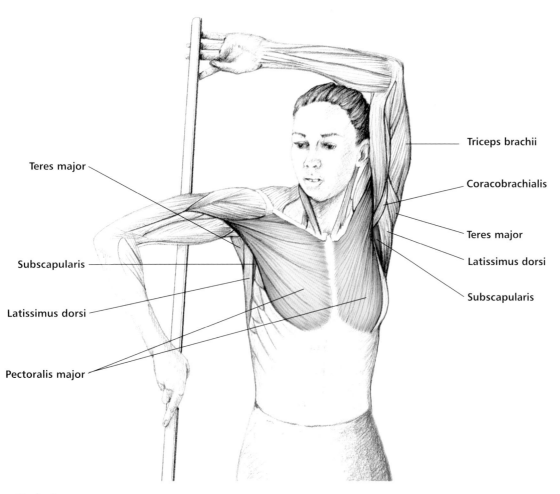

Triceps brachii

Coracobrachialis

Teres major

Latissimus dorsi

Subscapularis

Teres major

Subscapularis

Latissimus dorsi

Pectoralis major

Technique
Stand with your arm out and your forearm pointing downwards at 90 degrees. Place a broomstick in your hand and behind your elbow. With your other hand pull the top of the broomstick forward.

Muscles being stretched
Primary muscle: Subscapularis.
Secondary muscle: Pectoralis major.

Sports that benefit from this stretch
Martial arts. Tennis. Badminton. Squash. Rowing. Canoeing. Kayaking. Swimming. Cricket. Baseball. Athletics throwing field events. Wrestling.

Sports injury where stretch may be useful
Dislocation. Subluxation. Acromioclavicular separation. Sternoclavicular separation. Impingement syndrome. Rotator cuff tendonitis. Shoulder bursitis. Frozen shoulder (adhesive capsulitis).

Common problems and additional information for performing this stretch correctly
Many people are very tight in the rotator cuff muscles of the shoulder. Perform this stretch very slowly to start with and use extreme caution at all times.

Complementary stretch
019.

022: KNEELING FOREARM STRETCH

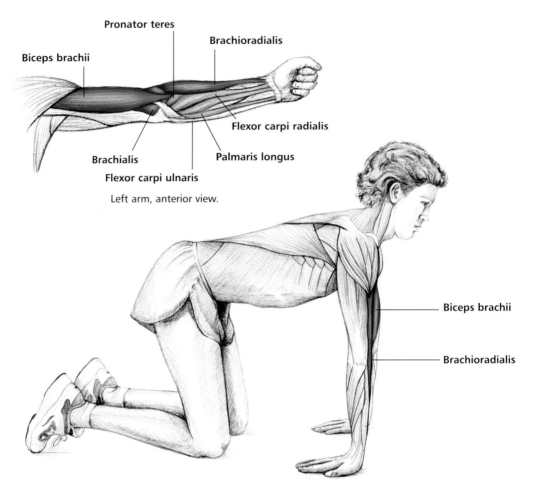

Pronator teres
Brachioradialis
Biceps brachii
Flexor carpi radialis
Palmaris longus
Brachialis
Flexor carpi ulnaris

Left arm, anterior view.

Biceps brachii
Brachioradialis

Technique
While crouching on your knees with your forearms facing forward and hands pointing backwards, slowly move rearward.

Muscles being stretched
Primary muscles: Biceps brachii. Brachialis. Brachioradialis.
Secondary muscles: Pronator teres. Flexor carpi radialis. Flexor carpi ulnaris. Palmaris longus.

Sports that benefit from this stretch
Basketball. Netball. Cricket. Baseball. Softball. Ice hockey. Field hockey. Martial arts. Tennis. Badminton. Squash. Rowing. Canoeing. Kayaking. Swimming. Athletics throwing field events. Volleyball. Wrestling.

Sports injury where stretch may be useful
Biceps tendon rupture. Bicepital tendonitis. Biceps strain. Elbow strain. Elbow dislocation. Elbow bursitis. Tennis elbow. Golfer's elbow. Thrower's elbow.

Common problems and additional information for performing this stretch correctly
Depending on where your muscles are most tight, you may feel this stretch more in your forearms or more in your upper arms. To make this stretch easier, move your hands towards your knees.

Complementary stretch
023.

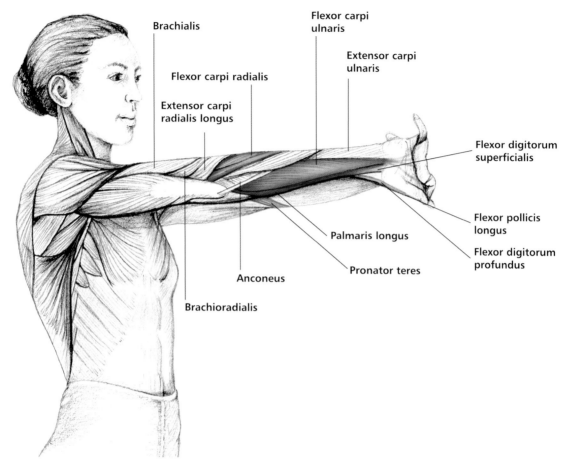

Brachialis

Flexor carpi ulnaris

Flexor carpi radialis

Extensor carpi ulnaris

Extensor carpi radialis longus

Flexor digitorum superficialis

Flexor pollicis longus

Flexor digitorum profundus

Palmaris longus

Pronator teres

Anconeus

Brachioradialis

Technique
Interlock your fingers in front of your chest and then straighten your arms and turn the palms of your hands outwards.

Muscles being stretched
Primary muscles: Pronator teres. Flexor carpi radialis. Flexor carpi ulnaris. Palmaris longus.
Secondary muscles: Flexor digitorum superficialis. Flexor digitorum profundus. Flexor pollicis longus.

Sports that benefit from this stretch
Basketball. Netball. Cricket. Baseball. Softball. Ice hockey. Field hockey. Martial arts. Tennis. Badminton. Squash. Rowing. Canoeing. Kayaking. Swimming. Athletics throwing field events. Volleyball. Wrestling.

Sports injury where stretch may be useful
Tennis elbow. Golfer's elbow. Thrower's elbow. Wrist sprain. Wrist dislocation. Wrist tendonitis. Carpel tunnel syndrome. Ulnar tunnel syndrome.

Common problems and additional information for performing this stretch correctly
The forearms, wrists and fingers comprise a multitude of small muscles, tendons and ligaments. Do not over stretch this area by applying too much force too quickly.

Complementary stretch
024.

024: FINGERS-DOWN FOREARM STRETCH

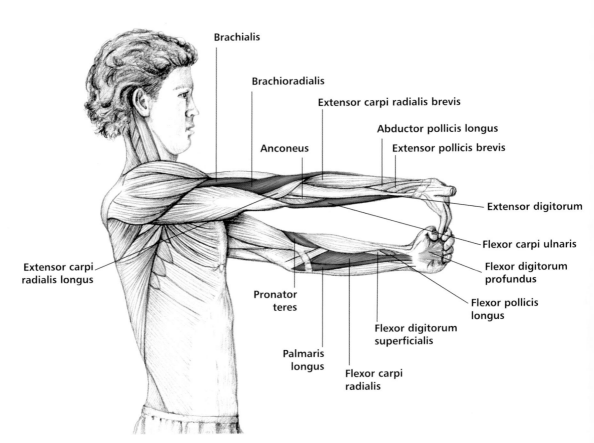

Brachialis

Brachioradialis

Extensor carpi radialis brevis

Abductor pollicis longus

Extensor pollicis brevis

Anconeus

Extensor digitorum

Flexor carpi ulnaris

Extensor carpi radialis longus

Flexor digitorum profundus

Pronator teres

Flexor pollicis longus

Flexor digitorum superficialis

Palmaris longus

Flexor carpi radialis

Technique
Hold onto your fingers and turn your palms outwards. Straighten your arm and then pull your fingers back using your other hand.

Muscles being stretched
Primary muscles: Brachialis. Brachioradialis. Pronator teres. Flexor carpi radialis. Flexor carpi ulnaris. Palmaris longus.
Secondary muscles: Flexor digitorum superficialis. Flexor digitorum profundus. Flexor pollicis longus.

Sports that benefit from this stretch
Basketball. Netball. Cricket. Baseball. Softball. Ice hockey. Field hockey. Martial arts. Tennis. Badminton. Squash. Rowing. Canoeing. Kayaking. Swimming. Athletics throwing field events. Volleyball. Wrestling.

Sports injury where stretch may be useful
Tennis elbow. Golfer's elbow. Thrower's elbow. Wrist sprain. Wrist dislocation. Wrist tendonitis. Carpel tunnel syndrome. Ulnar tunnel syndrome.

Common problems and additional information for performing this stretch correctly
The forearms, wrists and fingers comprise a multitude of small muscles, tendons and ligaments. Do not over stretch this area by applying too much force too quickly.

Complementary stretch
022.

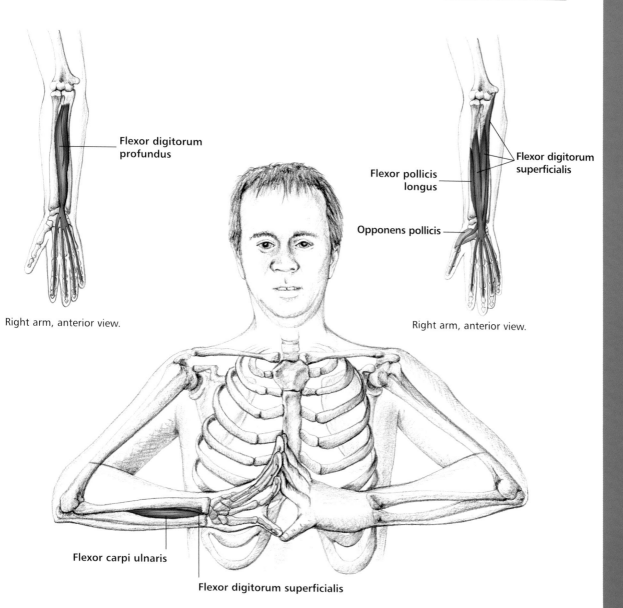

Flexor digitorum profundus

Flexor pollicis longus

Flexor digitorum superficialis

Opponens pollicis

Right arm, anterior view.

Right arm, anterior view.

Flexor carpi ulnaris

Flexor digitorum superficialis

Technique
Place the tips of your fingers together and push your palms towards each other.

Muscles being stretched
Primary muscles: Flexor digitorum superficialis. Flexor digitorum profundus. Flexor pollicis longus.
Secondary muscle: Opponens pollicis.

Sports that benefit from this stretch
Basketball. Netball. Cricket. Baseball. Softball. Ice hockey. Field hockey. Martial arts. Tennis. Badminton. Squash. Rowing. Canoeing. Kayaking. Swimming. Athletics field events. Volleyball. Wrestling.

Sports injury where stretch may be useful
Tennis elbow. Golfer's elbow. Thrower's elbow. Wrist sprain. Wrist dislocation. Wrist tendonitis. Carpel tunnel syndrome. Ulnar tunnel syndrome.

Common problems and additional information for performing this stretch correctly
The forearms, wrists and fingers comprise a multitude of small muscles, tendons and ligaments. Do not over stretch this area by applying too much force too quickly.

Complementary stretch
024.

026: FINGERS-DOWN WRIST STRETCH

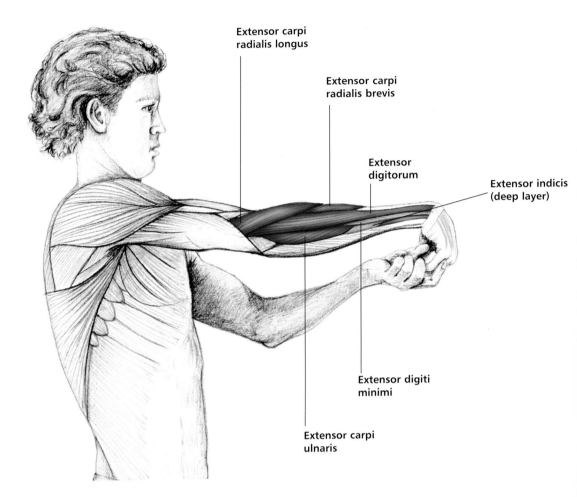

Extensor carpi
radialis longus

Extensor carpi
radialis brevis

Extensor
digitorum

Extensor indicis
(deep layer)

Extensor digiti
minimi

Extensor carpi
ulnaris

Technique
Hold on to your fingers while straightening your arm. Pull your fingers towards your body.

Muscles being stretched
Primary muscles: Extensor carpi ulnaris. Extensor carpi radialis longus and brevis. Extensor digitorum.
Secondary muscles: Extensor digiti minimi. Extensor indicis.

Sports that benefit from this stretch
Basketball. Netball. Cricket. Baseball. Softball. Ice hockey. Field hockey. Martial arts. Tennis. Badminton. Squash. Rowing. Canoeing. Kayaking. Swimming. Athletics throwing field events. Volleyball. Wrestling.

Sports injury where stretch may be useful
Tennis elbow. Golfer's elbow. Thrower's elbow. Wrist sprain. Wrist dislocation. Wrist tendonitis. Carpel tunnel syndrome. Ulnar tunnel syndrome.

Common problems and additional information for performing this stretch correctly
The forearms, wrists and fingers comprise a multitude of small muscles, tendons and ligaments. Do not over stretch this area by applying too much force too quickly.

Complementary stretch
027.

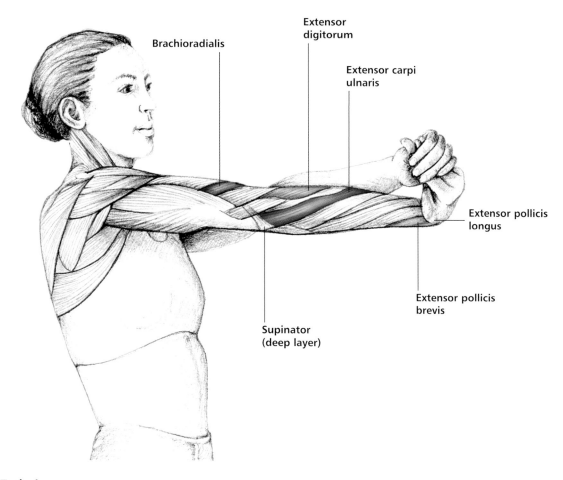

Brachioradialis

Extensor digitorum

Extensor carpi ulnaris

Extensor pollicis longus

Extensor pollicis brevis

Supinator (deep layer)

Technique
Place one arm straight out in front and parallel to the ground. Rotate your wrist down and outwards and then use your other hand to further rotate your hand upwards.

Muscles being stretched
Primary muscles: Brachioradialis. Extensor carpi ulnaris. Supinator.
Secondary muscles: Extensor digitorum. Extensor pollicis longus and brevis.

Sports that benefit from this stretch
Basketball. Netball. Cricket. Baseball. Softball. Ice hockey. Field hockey. Martial arts. Tennis. Badminton. Squash. Rowing. Canoeing. Kayaking. Swimming. Athletics throwing field events. Volleyball. Wrestling.

Sports injury where stretch may be useful
Tennis elbow. Golfer's elbow. Thrower's elbow. Wrist sprain. Wrist dislocation. Wrist tendonitis. Carpel tunnel syndrome. Ulnar tunnel syndrome.

Common problems and additional information for performing this stretch correctly
The forearms, wrists and fingers comprise a multitude of small muscles, tendons and ligaments. Do not over stretch this area by applying too much force too quickly.

Complementary stretch
026.

8

Stretches for the Stomach

028: ON ELBOWS STOMACH STRETCH

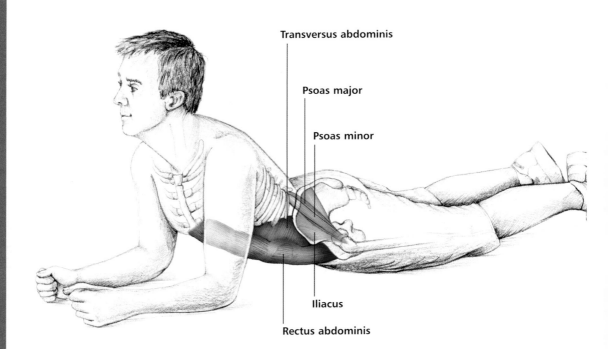

Transversus abdominis

Psoas major

Psoas minor

Iliacus

Rectus abdominis

Technique
Lie face down and bring your hands close to your shoulders. Keep your hips on the ground, look forward and rise up onto your elbows.

Muscles being stretched
Primary muscles: Transversus abdominis. Rectus abdominis.
Secondary muscles: Psoas major and minor. Iliacus.

Sports that benefit from this stretch
Basketball. Netball. Cricket. Baseball. Softball. Boxing. Golf. Hiking. Backpacking. Mountaineering. Orienteering. Ice hockey. Field hockey. Ice-skating. Roller-skating. Inline skating. Martial arts. Rowing. Canoeing. Kayaking. Running. Track. Cross-country. American football (gridiron). Soccer. Rugby. Snow skiing. Water skiing. Surfing. Walking. Race walking. Wrestling.

Sports injury where stretch may be useful
Abdominal muscle strain.

Common problems and additional information for performing this stretch correctly
For most people who spend their day in a seated position, (office workers, drivers, etc.) the muscles in the front of the body can become extremely tight and inflexible. Exercise caution when performing this stretch for the first time and allow plenty of rest time between each repetition.

Complementary stretch
030.

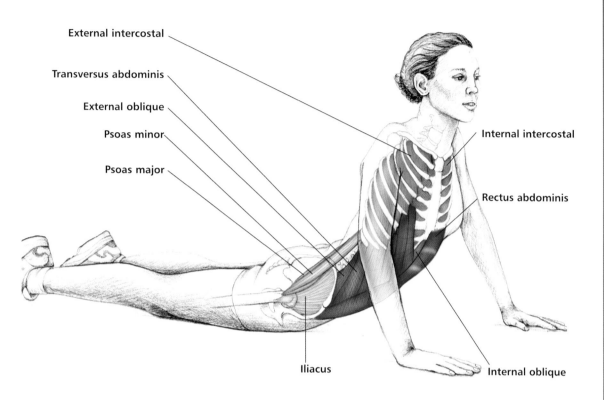

External intercostal

Transversus abdominis

External oblique

Psoas minor

Psoas major

Internal intercostal

Rectus abdominis

Iliacus

Internal oblique

Technique
Lie face down and bring your hands close to your shoulders. Keep your hips on the ground, look forward and rise up by straightening your arms.

Muscles being stretched
Primary muscles: External and internal intercostals. External and internal obliques. Transversus abdominis. Rectus abdominis.
Secondary muscles: Psoas major and minor. Iliacus.

Sports that benefit from this stretch
Basketball. Netball. Cricket. Baseball. Softball. Boxing. Golf. Hiking. Backpacking. Mountaineering. Orienteering. Ice hockey. Field hockey. Ice-skating. Roller-skating. Inline skating. Martial arts. Rowing. Canoeing. Kayaking. Running. Track. Cross-country. American football (gridiron). Soccer. Rugby. Snow skiing. Water skiing. Surfing. Walking. Race walking. Wrestling.

Sports injury where stretch may be useful
Abdominal muscle strain. Hip flexor strain. Iliopsoas tendonitis.

Common problems and additional information for performing this stretch correctly
For most people who spend their day in a seated position, (office workers, drivers, etc.) the muscles in the front of the body can become extremely tight and inflexible. Exercise caution when performing this stretch for the first time and allow plenty of rest time between each repetition.

Complementary stretch
030.

030: ROTATING STOMACH STRETCH

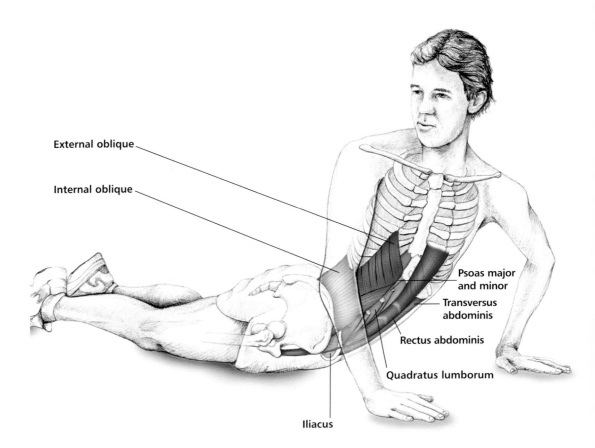

External oblique

Internal oblique

Psoas major and minor

Transversus abdominis

Rectus abdominis

Quadratus lumborum

Iliacus

Technique
Lie face down and bring your hands close to your shoulders. Keep your hips on the ground, look forward and rise up by straightening your arms. Then slowly bend one arm and rotate that shoulder towards the ground.

Muscles being stretched
Primary muscles: External and internal obliques. Transversus abdominis. Rectus abdominis.
Secondary muscles: Quadratus lumborum. Psoas major and minor. Iliacus.

Sports that benefit from this stretch
Basketball. Netball. Cricket. Baseball. Softball. Boxing. Golf. Hiking. Backpacking. Mountaineering. Orienteering. Ice hockey. Field hockey. Ice-skating. Roller-skating. Inline skating. Martial arts. Rowing. Canoeing. Kayaking. Running. Track. Cross-country. American football (gridiron). Soccer. Rugby. Snow skiing. Water skiing. Surfing. Walking. Race walking. Wrestling.

Sports injury where stretch may be useful
Abdominal muscle strain. Hip flexor strain. Iliopsoas tendonitis.

Common problems and additional information for performing this stretch correctly
For most people who spend their day in a seated position, (office workers, drivers, etc.) the muscles in the front of the body can become extremely tight and inflexible. Exercise caution when performing this stretch for the first time and allow plenty of rest time between each repetition.

Complementary stretch
031.

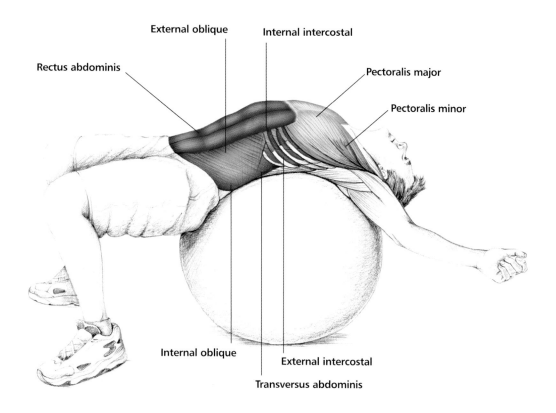

Technique
Sit on a Swiss ball and slowly roll the ball forward while leaning back. Allow your back and shoulders to rest on the ball and your arms to hang to each side.

Muscles being stretched
Primary muscles: External and internal intercostals. External and internal obliques. Transversus abdominis. Rectus abdominis.
Secondary muscles: Pectoralis major and minor.

Sports that benefit from this stretch
Basketball. Netball. Cricket. Baseball. Softball. Boxing. Golf. Hiking. Backpacking. Mountaineering. Orienteering. Ice hockey. Field hockey. Ice-skating. Roller-skating. Inline skating. Martial arts. Rowing. Canoeing. Kayaking. Running. Track. Cross-country. American football (gridiron). Soccer. Rugby. Snow skiing. Water skiing. Surfing. Walking. Race walking. Wrestling.

Sports injury where stretch may be useful
Abdominal muscle strain. Chest strain. Pectoral muscle insertion inflammation.

Common problems and additional information for performing this stretch correctly
For most people who spend their day in a seated position, (office workers, drivers, etc.) the muscles in the front of the body can become extremely tight and inflexible. Exercise caution when performing this stretch for the first time and allow plenty of rest time between each repetition.

Complementary stretch
029.

9

Stretches for the Back and Sides
(Upper, Middle, and Lower)

032: REACHING UPPER BACK STRETCH

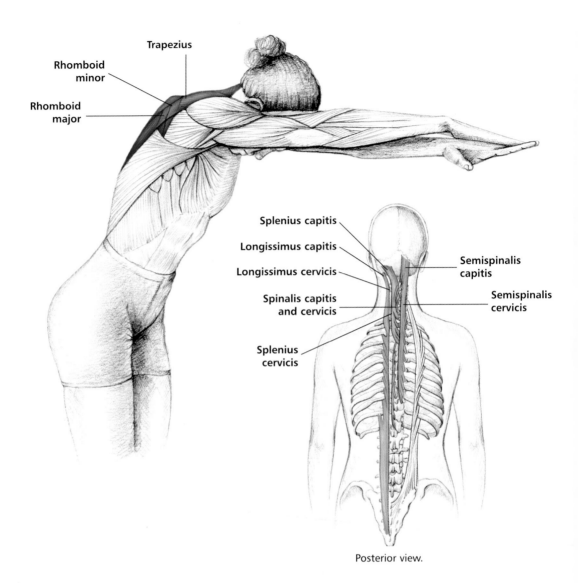

Posterior view.

Technique
Stand with your arms out in front and crossed over. Push your hands forward as far as possible and let your head fall forward.

Muscles being stretched
Primary muscles: Trapezius. Rhomboids.
Secondary muscles: Semispinalis capitis and cervicis. Spinalis capitis and cervicis. Longissimus capitis and cervicis. Splenius capitis and cervicis.

Sports that benefit from this stretch
Archery. Boxing. Cycling. Golf. Tennis. Badminton. Squash. Rowing. Canoeing. Kayaking. Snow skiing. Water skiing. Swimming.

Sports injury where stretch may be useful
Neck muscle strain. Whiplash (neck sprain). Cervical nerve stretch syndrome. Wryneck (acute torticollis). Upper back muscle strain. Upper back ligament sprain.

Additional information for performing this stretch correctly
Concentrate on reaching forward with your hands and separating your shoulder blades.

Complementary stretch
035.

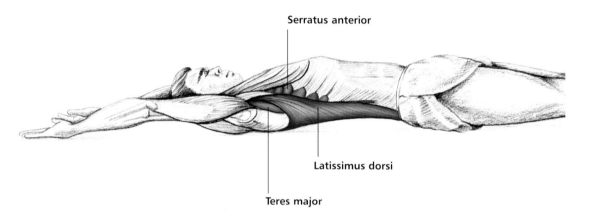

Serratus anterior

Latissimus dorsi

Teres major

Technique
Lie on your back and extend your arms behind you. Raise your toes and then lengthen your body as much as you can.

Muscles being stretched
Primary muscles: Serratus anterior. Latissimus dorsi.
Secondary muscle: Teres major.

Sports that benefit from this stretch
Basketball. Netball. Swimming. Volleyball.

Sports injury where stretch may be useful
Back muscle strain. Back ligament sprain.

Additional information for performing this stretch correctly
Concentrate on extending your legs by pushing with your heels, rather than your toes.

Complementary stretch
034.

034: REACH-UP BACK STRETCH

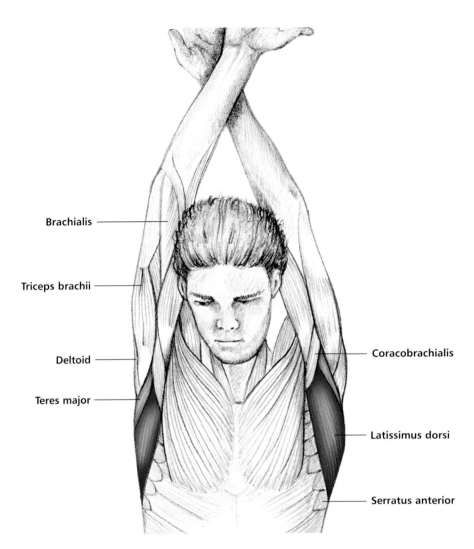

Brachialis

Triceps brachii

Deltoid

Teres major

Coracobrachialis

Latissimus dorsi

Serratus anterior

Technique
Stand with your arms crossed over and then raise them above your head. Reach up as far as you can.

Muscles being stretched
Primary muscle: Latissimus dorsi.
Secondary muscle: Teres major.

Sports that benefit from this stretch
Basketball. Netball. Swimming. Volleyball.

Sports injury where stretch may be useful
Neck muscle strain. Whiplash (neck sprain). Cervical nerve stretch syndrome. Wryneck (acute torticollis). Upper back muscle strain. Upper back ligament sprain.

Additional information for performing this stretch correctly
Let your head fall forward so that your arms can reach straight upwards without touching your head.

Complementary stretch
033.

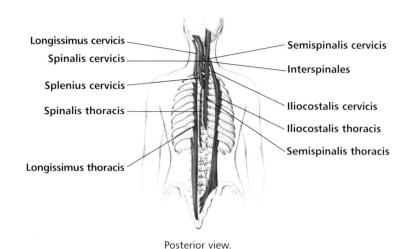

Longissimus cervicis
Spinalis cervicis
Splenius cervicis
Spinalis thoracis
Longissimus thoracis

Semispinalis cervicis
Interspinales
Iliocostalis cervicis
Iliocostalis thoracis
Semispinalis thoracis

Posterior view.

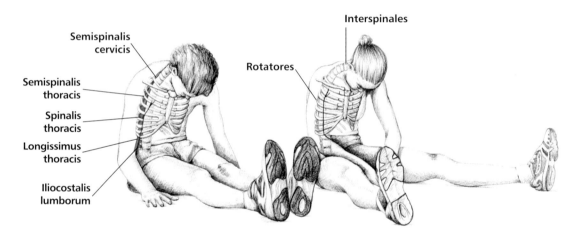

Semispinalis cervicis
Semispinalis thoracis
Spinalis thoracis
Longissimus thoracis
Iliocostalis lumborum

Rotatores

Interspinales

Technique
Sit on the ground with your legs straight out in front or at 45 degrees apart. Keep your toes pointing upwards and rest your arms by your side or on your lap. Relax your back and neck and then let your head and chest fall forward.

Muscles being stretched
Primary muscles: Semispinalis cervicis and thoracis. Spinalis cervicis and thoracis. Longissimus cervicis and thoracis. Splenius cervicis. Iliocostalis cervicis and thoracis. Secondary muscles: Interspinales. Rotatores.

Sports that benefit from this stretch
Cricket. Baseball. Softball. American football (gridiron). Rugby. Cycling. Golf. Hiking. Backpacking. Mountaineering. Orienteering. Ice hockey. Field hockey. Tennis. Badminton. Squash. Rowing. Canoeing. Kayaking. Swimming.

Sports injury where stretch may be useful
Neck muscle strain. Whiplash (neck sprain). Cervical nerve stretch syndrome. Wryneck (acute torticollis). Back muscle strain. Back ligament sprain.

Common problems and additional information for performing this stretch correctly
Where this stretch is primarily felt will depend on where you are most tight. Some people will feel most tension in the neck and upper back, whereas others will feel most tension in the lower back and hamstrings. This stretch gives a good indication of where you need to improve your flexibility.

Complementary stretch
032.

036: SITTING SIDE REACH STRETCH

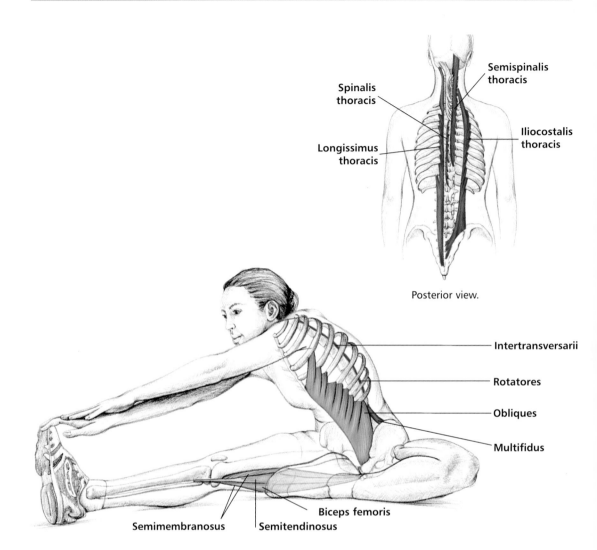

Spinalis
thoracis

Semispinalis
thoracis

Iliocostalis
thoracis

Longissimus
thoracis

Posterior view.

Intertransversarii

Rotatores

Obliques

Multifidus

Biceps femoris

Semimembranosus   Semitendinosus

Technique
Sit with one leg straight out to the side and your toes pointing up. Then bring your other foot up to your knee and let your head fall forward. Reach towards the outside of your toes with both hands.

Muscles being stretched
Primary muscles: Semispinalis thoracis. Spinalis thoracis. Longissimus thoracis. Iliocostalis thoracis. Iliocostalis lumborum. Inter-transversarii. Rotatores. Multifidus.
Secondary muscles: Obliques. Semi-membranosus. Semitendinosus. Biceps femoris.

Sports that benefit from this stretch
Cricket. Baseball. Softball. Boxing. American football (gridiron). Rugby. Cycling. Golf. Hiking. Backpacking. Mountaineering. Orienteering. Ice hockey. Field hockey. Tennis. Badminton. Squash. Rowing. Canoeing. Kayaking. Swimming. Running. Walking. Race walking.

Sports injury where stretch may be useful
Neck muscle strain. Whiplash (neck sprain). Cervical nerve stretch syndrome. Wryneck (acute torticollis). Back muscle strain. Back ligament sprain.

Additional information for performing this stretch correctly
It is not important to be able to touch your toes. Simply reaching towards the outside of your toes is sufficient.

Complementary stretch
049.

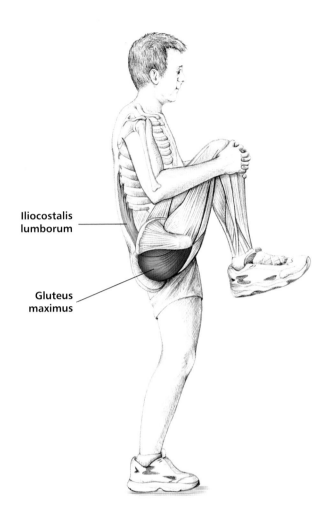

Iliocostalis
lumborum

Gluteus
maximus

Technique
While standing, use your hands to bring one knee into your chest.

Muscles being stretched
Primary muscle: Gluteus maximus.
Secondary muscle: Iliocostalis lumborum.

Sports that benefit from this stretch
Basketball. Netball. Cycling. Hiking. Backpacking. Mountaineering. Orienteering. Ice hockey. Field hockey. Ice-skating. Roller-skating. Inline skating. Martial arts. Running. Track. Cross-country. American football (gridiron). Soccer. Rugby. Snow skiing. Water skiing. Surfing. Walking. Race walking.

Sports injury where stretch may be useful
Lower back muscle strain. Lower back ligament sprain. Hamstring strain.

Additional information for performing this stretch correctly
Make sure you have good balance when performing this stretch, or lean against an object to stop yourself from falling over.

Complementary stretch
038.

038: LYING KNEE-TO-CHEST STRETCH

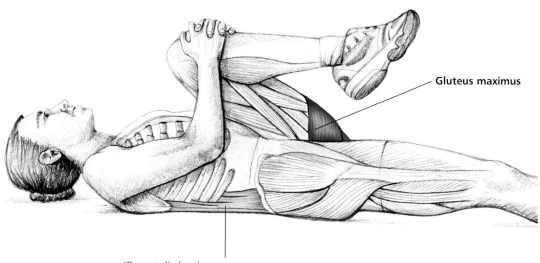

Gluteus maximus

Iliocostalis lumborum

Technique
Lie on your back and keep one leg flat on the ground. Use your hands to bring your other knee into your chest.

Muscles being stretched
Primary muscle: Gluteus maximus.
Secondary muscle: Iliocostalis lumborum.

Sports that benefit from this stretch
Basketball. Netball. Cycling. Hiking. Backpacking. Mountaineering. Orienteering. Ice hockey. Field hockey. Ice-skating. Roller-skating. Inline skating. Martial arts. Running. Track. Cross-country. American football (gridiron). Soccer. Rugby. Snow skiing. Water skiing. Surfing. Walking. Race walking.

Sports injury where stretch may be useful
Lower back muscle strain. Lower back ligament sprain. Hamstring strain.

Additional information for performing this stretch correctly
Rest your back, head and neck on the ground and do not be tempted to raise your head off the ground.

Complementary stretch
039.

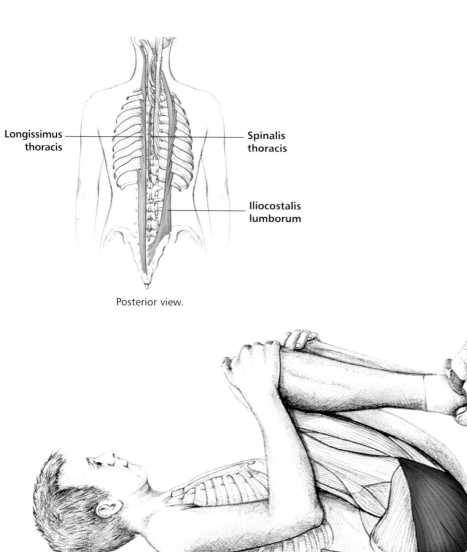

Longissimus thoracis
Spinalis thoracis
Iliocostalis lumborum

Posterior view.

Iliocostalis lumborum
Gluteus maximus

Technique
Lie on your back and use your hands to bring both knees into your chest.

Muscles being stretched
Primary muscle: Gluteus maximus.
Secondary muscles: Iliocostalis lumborum. Spinalis thoracis. Longissimus thoracis.

Sports that benefit from this stretch
Basketball. Netball. Cycling. Hiking. Backpacking. Mountaineering. Orienteering. Ice hockey. Field hockey. Ice-skating. Roller-skating. Inline skating. Martial arts. Running. Track. Cross-country. American football (gridiron). Soccer. Rugby. Snow skiing. Water skiing. Surfing. Walking. Race walking.

Sports injury where stretch may be useful
Lower back muscle strain. Lower back ligament sprain. Hamstring strain.

Additional information for performing this stretch correctly
Rest your back, head and neck on the ground and don't be tempted to raise your head off the ground.

Complementary stretch
037.

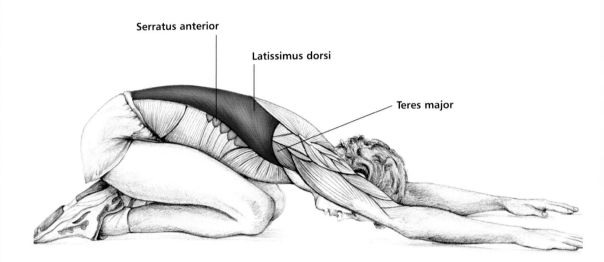

Serratus anterior

Latissimus dorsi

Teres major

Technique
Kneel on the ground and reach forward with your hands. Let your head fall forward and push your buttocks towards your feet.

Muscles being stretched
Primary muscle: Latissimus dorsi.
Secondary muscles: Teres major. Serratus anterior.

Sports that benefit from this stretch
Basketball. Netball. Swimming. Volleyball.

Sports injury where stretch may be useful
Lower back muscle strain. Lower back ligament sprain.

Additional information for performing this stretch correctly
Use your hands and fingers to walk your arms forward and extend this stretch, but do not lift your backside off your feet.

Complementary stretch
033.

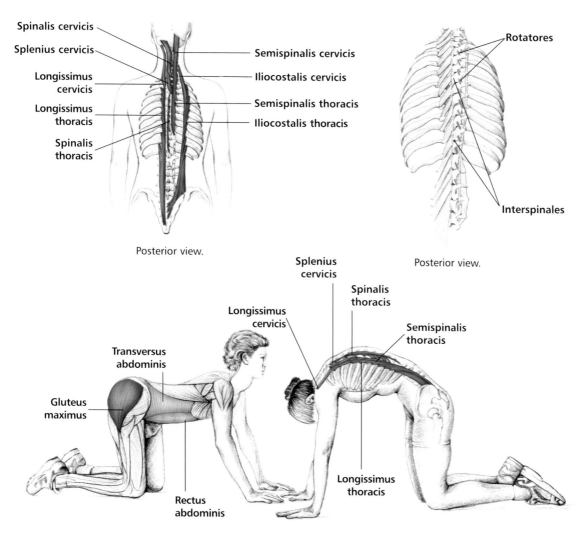

Posterior view.

Posterior view.

Technique
Kneel on your hands and knees. Look up and let your back slump downwards. Then let your head fall forward and arch your back upwards.

Muscles being stretched
Back slumping downwards
Primary muscle: Gluteus maximus.
Secondary muscles: Transversus abdominis. Rectus abdominis.
Back arching upwards
Primary muscles: Semispinalis cervicis and thoracis. Spinalis cervicis and thoracis. Longissimus cervicis and thoracis. Splenius cervicis. Iliocostalis cervicis and thoracis.
Secondary muscles: Interspinales. Rotatores.

Sports that benefit from this stretch
Cricket. Baseball. Softball. Cycling. Golf. Hiking. Backpacking. Mountaineering. Orienteering. Ice hockey. Field hockey. Tennis. Badminton. Squash. Rowing. Canoeing. Swimming. Kayaking. Running. Track. Cross-country. American football (gridiron). Soccer. Rugby. Walking. Race walking.

Sports injury where stretch may be useful
Neck muscle strain. Whiplash (neck sprain). Cervical nerve stretch syndrome. Wryneck (acute torticollis). Back muscle strain. Back ligament sprain.

Additional information for performing this stretch correctly
Perform this stretch slowly and deliberately, resting your weight evenly on both your knees and hands.

Complementary stretches
035, 031.

042: KNEELING BACK ROTATION STRETCH

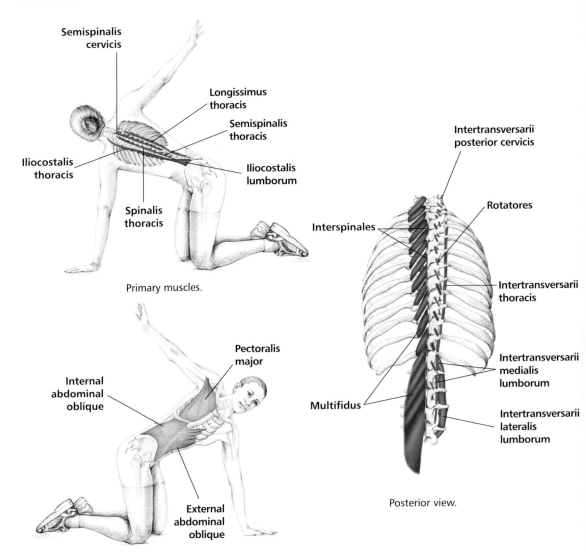

Primary muscles.

Secondary muscles.

Posterior view.

Technique
Kneel on the ground and raise one arm. Then rotate your shoulders and middle back while looking upwards.

Muscles being stretched
Primary muscles: Semispinalis thoracis. Spinalis thoracis. Longissimus thoracis. Iliocostalis thoracis. Iliocostalis lumborum. Multifidus. Rotatores. Intertransversarii. Interspinales.
Secondary muscles: External and internal obliques. Pectoralis major.

Sports that benefit from this stretch
Archery. Basketball. Netball. Cricket. Baseball. Softball. Boxing. Cycling. Golf. Hiking. Backpacking. Mountaineering. Orienteering. Ice hockey. Field hockey. Ice-skating. Roller-skating. Inline skating. Martial arts. Tennis. Badminton. Squash. Rowing. Canoeing. Kayaking. Running. Track. Cross-country. American football (gridiron). Soccer. Rugby. Snow skiing. Water skiing. Surfing. Swimming. Athletics field events. Walking. Race walking. Wrestling.

Sports injury where stretch may be useful
Back muscle strain. Back ligament sprain. Abdominal muscle strain (obliques).

Additional information for performing this stretch correctly
Keep your arm pointing straight upward and follow your hand with your eyes. This will help to further extend the stretch into your neck.

Complementary stretch
043.

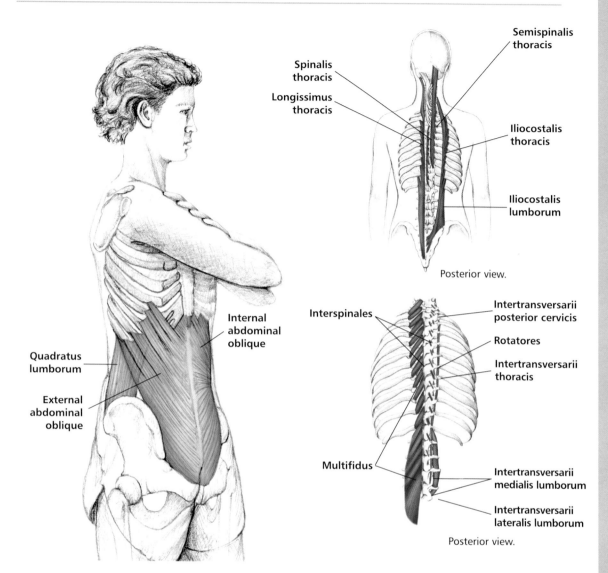

Posterior view.

Posterior view.

Technique
Stand with your feet shoulder-width apart. Place your hands across your chest while keeping your back and shoulders upright. Slowly rotate your shoulders to one side.

Muscles being stretched
Primary muscles: Semispinalis thoracis. Spinalis thoracis. Longissimus thoracis. Iliocostalis thoracis. Iliocostalis lumborum. Multifidus. Rotatores. Intertransversarii. Interspinales.
Secondary muscles: Quadratus lumborum. External and internal obliques.

Sports that benefit from this stretch
Archery. Basketball. Netball. Cricket. Baseball. Softball. Boxing. American football (gridiron). Rugby. Cycling. Golf. Hiking. Backpacking. Mountaineering. Orienteering. Ice hockey. Field hockey. Ice-skating. Roller-skating. Inline skating. Martial arts. Tennis. Badminton. Squash. Rowing. Canoeing. Kayaking. Water skiing. Surfing. Swimming. Running. Track. Cross-country. Soccer. Snow skiing. Athletic field events. Walking. Race walking. Wrestling.

Sports injury where stretch may be useful
Back muscle strain. Back ligament sprain. Abdominal muscle strain (obliques).

Additional information for performing this stretch correctly
To further extend this stretch use your hands to pull your upper body further around.

Complementary stretch
045.

044: STANDING REACH-UP BACK ROTATION STRETCH

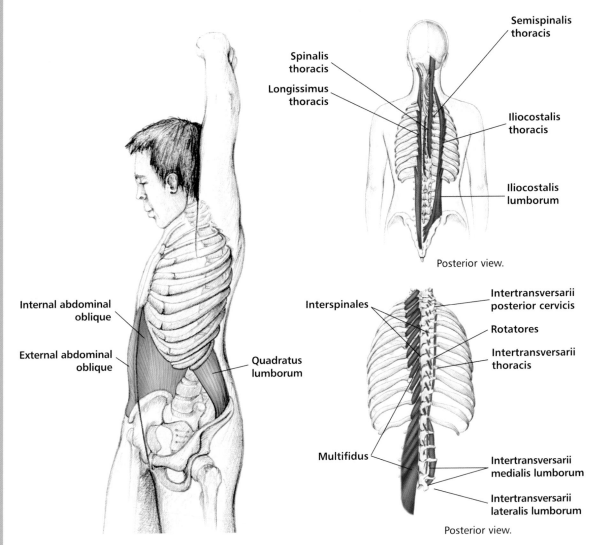

Posterior view.

Posterior view.

Technique
Stand with your feet shoulder-width apart. Place your hands above your head while keeping your back and shoulders upright. Slowly rotate your shoulders to one side.

Muscles being stretched
Primary muscles: Semispinalis thoracis. Spinalis thoracis. Longissimus thoracis. Iliocostalis thoracis. Iliocostalis lumborum. Multifidus. Rotatores. Intertransversarii. Interspinales. Secondary muscles: Quadratus lumborum. External and internal obliques.

Sports that benefit from this stretch
Archery. Basketball. Netball. Cricket. Baseball. Softball. Boxing. American football (gridiron). Rugby. Cycling. Golf. Hiking. Backpacking. Mountaineering. Orienteering. Ice hockey. Field hockey. Ice-skating. Roller-skating. Inline skating. Martial arts. Tennis. Badminton. Squash. Rowing. Canoeing. Kayaking. Running. Track. Cross-country. Snow skiing. Water skiing. Surfing. Swimming. Athletics field events. Walking. Race walking. Wrestling.

Sports injury where stretch may be useful
Back muscle strain. Back ligament sprain. Abdominal muscle strain (obliques).

Common problems and additional information for performing this stretch correctly
Lean back slightly to emphasize the *oblique* muscles. Do not do this if you suffer from lower back pain.

Complementary stretch
042.

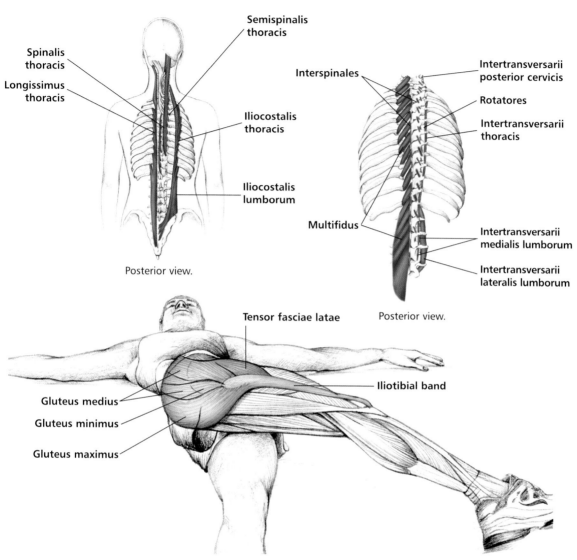

Posterior view.

Posterior view.

Technique
Lie on your back and cross one leg over the other. Keep your arms out to the side and both legs straight. Let your back and hips rotate with your leg.

Muscles being stretched
Primary muscles: Semispinalis thoracis. Spinalis thoracis. Longissimus thoracis. Iliocostalis thoracis. Iliocostalis lumborum. Multifidus. Rotatores. Intertransversarii. Interspinales. Secondary muscles: Gluteus maximus, medius and minimus. Tensor fasciae latae.

Sports that benefit from this stretch
Cycling. Hiking. Backpacking. Mountaineering. Orienteering. Ice hockey. Field hockey. Ice-skating. Roller-skating. Inline skating. Martial arts. Running. Track. Cross-country. American football (gridiron). Soccer. Rugby. Snow skiing. Water skiing. Surfing. Walking. Race walking. Wrestling.

Sports injury where stretch may be useful
Lower back muscle strain. Lower back ligament sprain. Iliotibial band syndrome.

Additional information for performing this stretch correctly
Keep your shoulders on the ground and avoid lifting them during this stretch. Do not throw your leg over to the side; simply let the weight of your leg do most of the stretching for you.

Complementary stretch
046.

046: LYING KNEE ROLL-OVER STRETCH

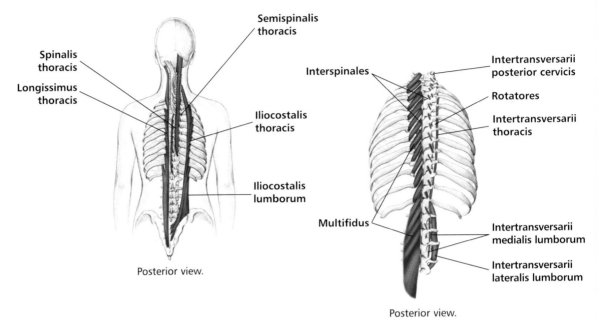

Semispinalis thoracis

Spinalis thoracis

Longissimus thoracis

Iliocostalis thoracis

Iliocostalis lumborum

Posterior view.

Interspinales

Intertransversarii posterior cervicis

Rotatores

Intertransversarii thoracis

Multifidus

Intertransversarii medialis lumborum

Intertransversarii lateralis lumborum

Posterior view.

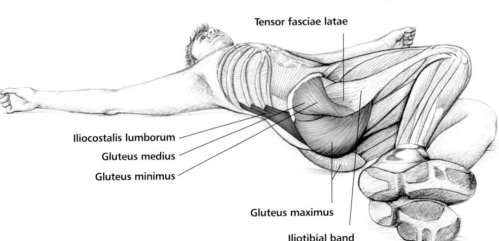

Tensor fasciae latae

Iliocostalis lumborum

Gluteus medius

Gluteus minimus

Gluteus maximus

Iliotibial band

Technique
Lie on your back, keep your knees together and raise them slightly. Keep your arms out to the side and then let your back and hips rotate with your knees.

Muscles being stretched
Primary muscles: Semispinalis thoracis. Spinalis thoracis. Longissimus thoracis. Iliocostalis thoracis. Iliocostalis lumborum. Multifidus. Rotatores. Intertransversarii. Interspinales. Secondary muscles: Gluteus maximus, medius and minimus.

Sports that benefit from this stretch
Cycling. Hiking. Backpacking. Mountaineering. Orienteering. Ice hockey. Field hockey. Ice-skating. Roller-skating. Inline skating. Martial arts. Running. Track. Cross-country. American football (gridiron). Soccer. Rugby. Snow skiing. Water skiing. Surfing. Walking. Race walking. Wrestling.

Sports injury where stretch may be useful
Lower back muscle strain. Lower back ligament sprain. Iliotibial band syndrome.

Additional information for performing this stretch correctly
Keep your shoulders on the ground and avoid lifting them during this stretch. Do not throw your legs over to the side; simply let the weight of your legs do most of the stretching for you.

Complementary stretch
043.

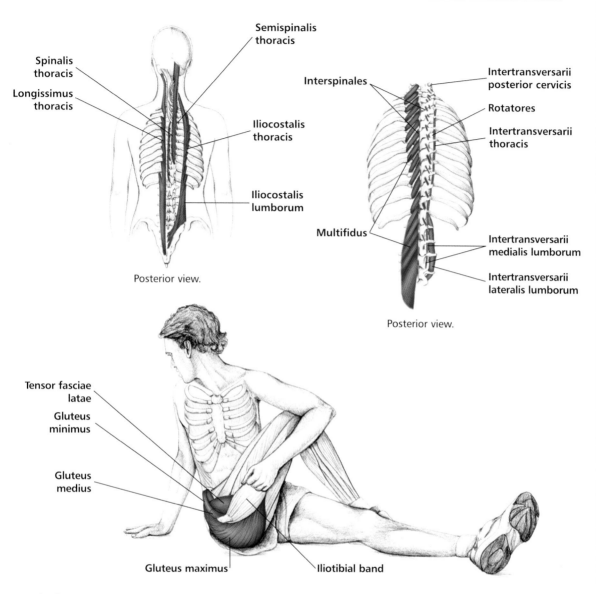

Posterior view.

Posterior view.

Technique
Sit with one leg straight and the other leg crossed over your knee. Turn your shoulders and put your arm onto your raised knee to help rotate your shoulders and back.

Muscles being stretched
Primary muscles: Gluteus maximus, medius and minimus. Tensor fasciae latae.
Secondary muscles: Semispinalis thoracis. Spinalis thoracis. Longissimus thoracis. Iliocostalis thoracis. Iliocostalis lumborum. Multifidus. Rotatores. Intertransversarii. Interspinales.

Sports that benefit from this stretch
Cycling. Hiking. Backpacking. Mountaineering. Orienteering. Ice hockey. Field hockey. Ice-skating. Roller-skating. Inline skating. Martial arts. Running. Track. Cross-country. American football (gridiron). Soccer. Rugby. Snow skiing. Water skiing. Walking. Race walking. Wrestling.

Sports injury where stretch may be useful
Lower back muscle strain. Lower back ligament sprain. Abdominal muscle strain (obliques). Iliotibial band syndrome.

Additional information for performing this stretch correctly
Keep your hips straight and concentrate on rotating your lower back.

Complementary stretch
045.

048: KNEELING REACH-AROUND STRETCH

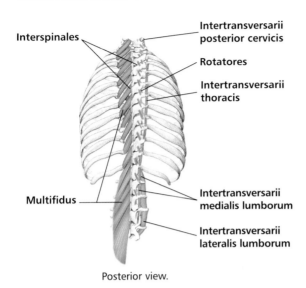

Interspinales

Intertransversarii posterior cervicis

Rotatores

Intertransversarii thoracis

Intertransversarii medialis lumborum

Intertransversarii lateralis lumborum

Multifidus

Posterior view.

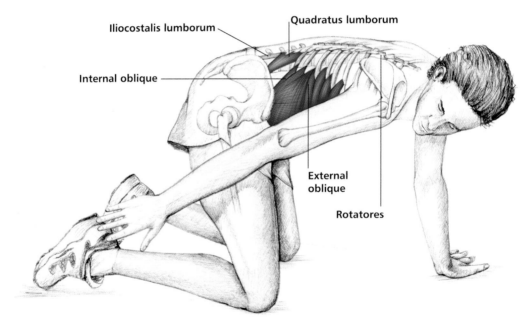

Iliocostalis lumborum

Quadratus lumborum

Internal oblique

External oblique

Rotatores

Technique
Kneel on your hands and knees and then take one hand and reach around towards your ankle. Keep your back parallel to the ground.

Muscles being stretched
Primary muscles: Quadratus lumborum. External and internal obliques.
Secondary muscles: Iliocostalis lumborum. Intertransversarii. Rotatores. Multifidus.

Sports that benefit from this stretch
Cricket. Baseball. Softball. Boxing. American football (gridiron). Rugby. Hiking. Backpacking. Mountaineering. Orienteering. Ice hockey. Field hockey. Martial arts. Rowing. Canoeing. Kayaking. Surfing. Wrestling.

Sports injury where stretch may be useful
Lower back muscle strain. Lower back ligament sprain. Abdominal muscle strain (obliques).

Additional information for performing this stretch correctly
Keep your thighs vertical, (straight up and down) and your back straight and parallel to the ground. Balance your weight evenly on both your knees and your hand.

Complementary stretch
050.

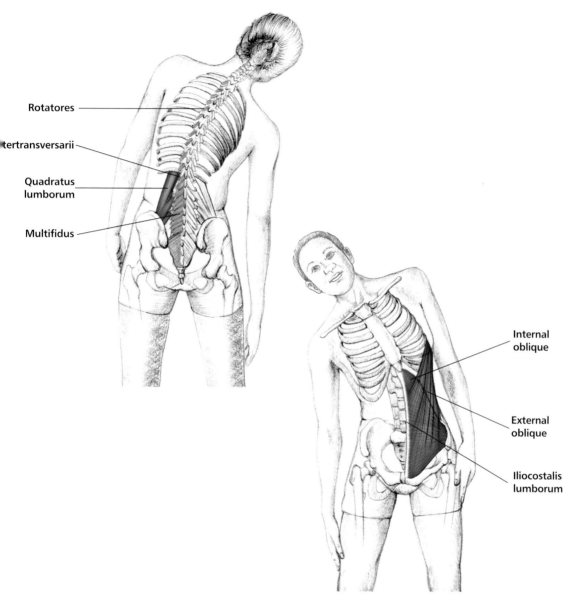

Rotatores

Intertransversarii

Quadratus lumborum

Multifidus

Internal oblique

External oblique

Iliocostalis lumborum

Technique
Stand with your feet about shoulder-width apart and look forward. Keep your body upright and slowly bend to the left or right. Reach down your leg with your hand and do not bend forward.

Muscles being stretched
Primary muscles: Quadratus lumborum. External and internal obliques.
Secondary muscles: Iliocostalis lumborum. Intertransversarii. Rotatores. Multifidus.

Sports that benefit from this stretch
Cricket. Baseball. Softball. Boxing. American football (gridiron). Rugby. Hiking. Backpacking. Mountaineering. Orienteering. Ice hockey. Field hockey. Martial arts. Rowing. Canoeing. Kayaking. Surfing. Wrestling.

Sports injury where stretch may be useful
Lower back muscle strain. Lower back ligament sprain. Abdominal muscle strain (obliques).

Common problems and additional information for performing this stretch correctly
Do not lean forward or backward: concentrate on keeping your upper body straight.

Complementary stretch
050.

050: SITTING LATERAL SIDE STRETCH

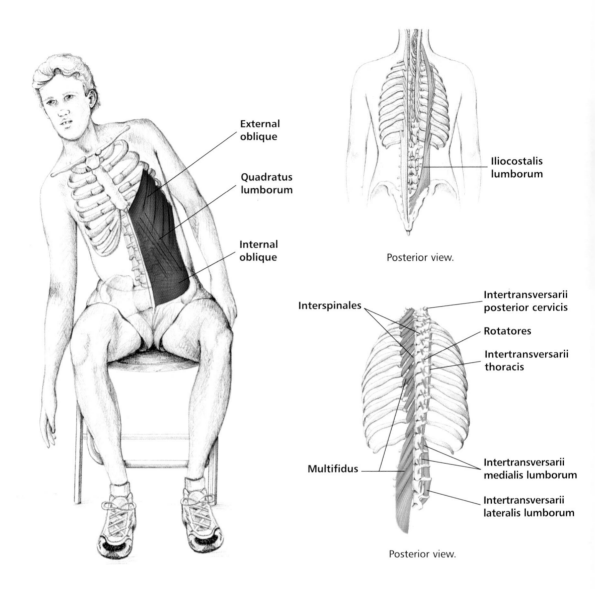

External oblique

Quadratus lumborum

Internal oblique

Iliocostalis lumborum

Posterior view.

Interspinales

Intertransversarii posterior cervicis

Rotatores

Intertransversarii thoracis

Multifidus

Intertransversarii medialis lumborum

Intertransversarii lateralis lumborum

Posterior view.

Technique

While sitting on a chair with your feet flat on the ground, look straight ahead and keep your body upright. Slowly bend to the left or right while reaching towards the ground with one hand. Do not bend forward.

Muscles being stretched

Primary muscles: Quadratus lumborum. External and internal obliques.
Secondary muscles: Iliocostalis lumborum. Intertransversarii. Rotatores. Multifidus.

Sports that benefit from this stretch

Cricket. Baseball. Softball. Boxing. American football (gridiron). Rugby. Hiking. Backpacking. Mountaineering. Orienteering. Ice hockey. Field hockey. Martial arts. Rowing. Canoeing. Kayaking. Surfing. Wrestling.

Sports injury where stretch may be useful

Lower back muscle strain. Lower back ligament sprain. Abdominal muscle strain (obliques).

Additional information for performing this stretch correctly

Do not lean forward or backward: concentrate on keeping your upper body straight.

Complementary stretch

036.

10 Stretches for the Hips and Buttocks

051: LYING CROSS-OVER KNEE PULL-DOWN STRETCH

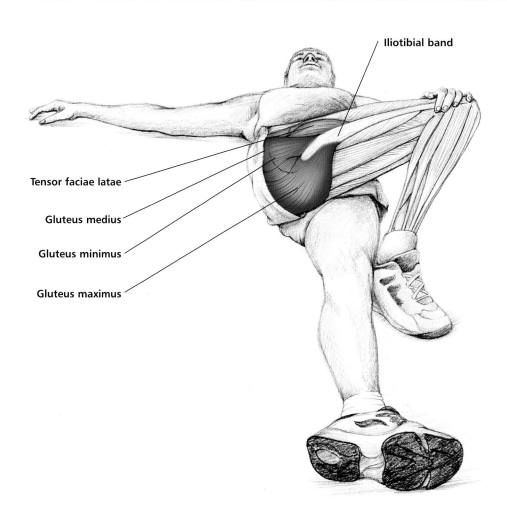

Iliotibial band

Tensor faciae latae

Gluteus medius

Gluteus minimus

Gluteus maximus

Technique
Lie on your back and cross one leg over the other. Bring your foot up to your opposite knee and with your opposite arm pull your raised knee towards the ground.

Muscles being stretched
Primary muscles: Gluteus medius and minimus.
Secondary muscle: Tensor fasciae latae.

Sports that benefit from this stretch
Cycling. Hiking. Backpacking. Mountaineering. Orienteering. Ice hockey. Field hockey. Ice-skating. Roller-skating. Inline skating. Martial arts. Running. Track. Cross-country. American football (gridiron). Soccer. Rugby. Snow skiing. Water skiing. Walking. Race walking.

Sports injury where stretch may be useful
Lower back muscle strain. Lower back ligament sprain. Iliotibial band syndrome.

Additional information for performing this stretch correctly
Keep your shoulders on the ground and concentrate on pulling your raised knee to the ground, not up towards your chest.

Complementary stretch
059.

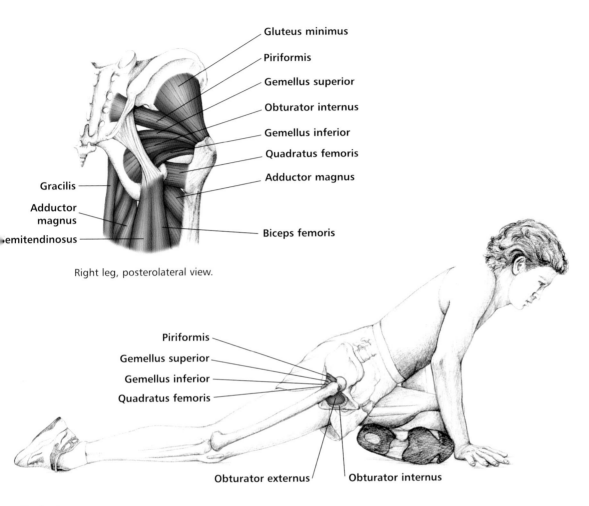

Gluteus minimus
Piriformis
Gemellus superior
Obturator internus
Gemellus inferior
Quadratus femoris
Adductor magnus
Biceps femoris

Gracilis
Adductor magnus
Semitendinosus

Right leg, posterolateral view.

Piriformis
Gemellus superior
Gemellus inferior
Quadratus femoris

Obturator externus
Obturator internus

Technique
Lie on your stomach and bend one leg under your stomach. Lean towards the ground.

Muscles being stretched
Primary muscle: Piriformis.
Secondary muscles: Gemellus superior and inferior. Obturator internus and externus. Quadratus femoris.

Sports that benefit from this stretch
Cycling. Hiking. Backpacking. Mountaineering. Orienteering. Ice hockey. Field hockey. Ice-skating. Roller-skating. Inline skating. Martial arts. Running. Track. Cross-country. American football (gridiron). Soccer. Rugby. Snow skiing. Water skiing. Walking. Race walking.

Sports injury where stretch may be useful
Piriformis syndrome. Snapping hip syndrome. Trochanteric bursitis.

Common problems and additional information for performing this stretch correctly
This position can be a little hard to get into, so make sure you are well supported and use your hands for balance.

Complementary stretch
054.

053: STANDING LEG TUCK HIP STRETCH

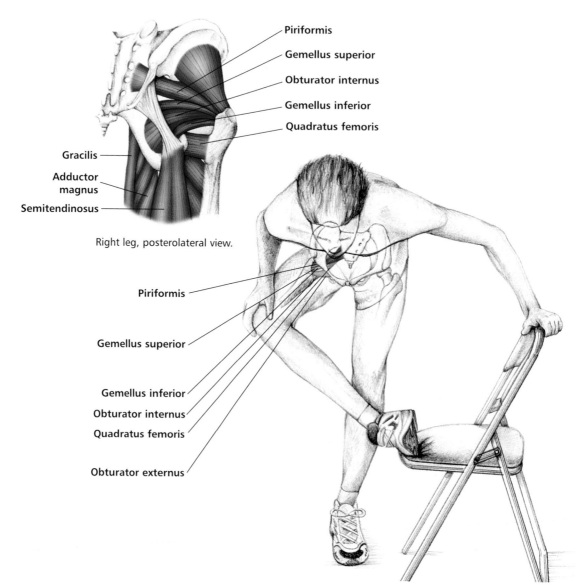

Right leg, posterolateral view.

Piriformis
Gemellus superior
Obturator internus
Gemellus inferior
Quadratus femoris
Gracilis
Adductor magnus
Semitendinosus

Piriformis
Gemellus superior
Gemellus inferior
Obturator internus
Quadratus femoris
Obturator externus

Technique
Stand beside a chair or table and place the foot furthest from the object onto the object. Relax your leg, lean forward and bend your other leg, lowering yourself towards the ground.

Muscles being stretched
Primary muscle: Piriformis.
Secondary muscles: Gemellus superior and inferior. Obturator internus and externus. Quadratus femoris.

Sports that benefit from this stretch
Cycling. Hiking. Backpacking. Mountaineering. Orienteering. Ice hockey. Field hockey. Ice-skating. Roller-skating. Inline skating. Martial arts. Running. Track. Cross-country. American football (gridiron). Soccer. Rugby. Snow skiing. Water skiing. Walking. Race walking.

Sports injury where stretch may be useful
Piriformis syndrome. Snapping hip syndrome. Trochanteric bursitis.

Common problems and additional information for performing this stretch correctly
Use the leg you are standing on to regulate the intensity of this stretch. The lower you go, the more tension you will feel.

Complementary stretch
052.

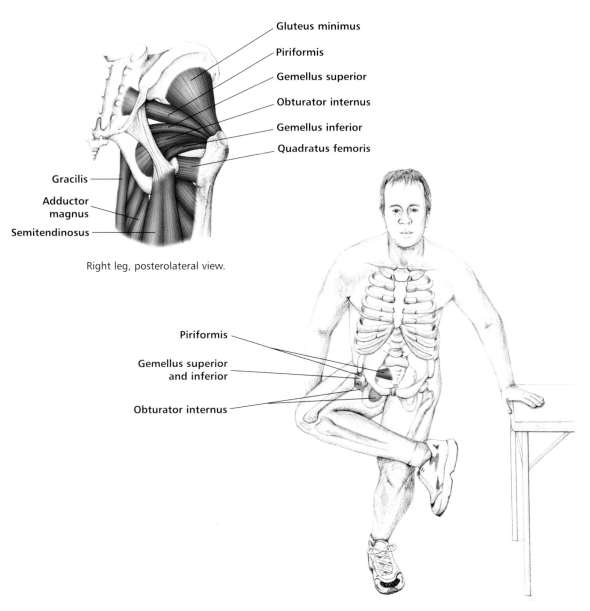

Gluteus minimus
Piriformis
Gemellus superior
Obturator internus
Gemellus inferior
Quadratus femoris

Gracilis
Adductor magnus
Semitendinosus

Right leg, posterolateral view.

Piriformis
Gemellus superior and inferior
Obturator internus

Technique
Stand beside a chair or table for balance, and place one ankle on your opposite knee. Slowly lower yourself towards the ground.

Muscles being stretched
Primary muscle: Piriformis.
Secondary muscles: Gemellus superior and inferior. Obturator internus and externus. Quadratus femoris.

Sports that benefit from this stretch
Cycling. Hiking. Backpacking. Mountaineering. Orienteering. Ice hockey. Field hockey. Ice-skating. Roller-skating. Inline skating. Martial arts. Running. Track. Cross-country. American football (gridiron). Soccer. Rugby. Snow skiing. Water skiing. Walking. Race walking.

Sports injury where stretch may be useful
Piriformis syndrome. Snapping hip syndrome. Trochanteric bursitis.

Common problems and additional information for performing this stretch correctly
Use the leg you are standing on to regulate the intensity of this stretch. The lower you go, the more tension you will feel.

Complementary stretch
060.

055: SITTING ROTATIONAL HIP STRETCH

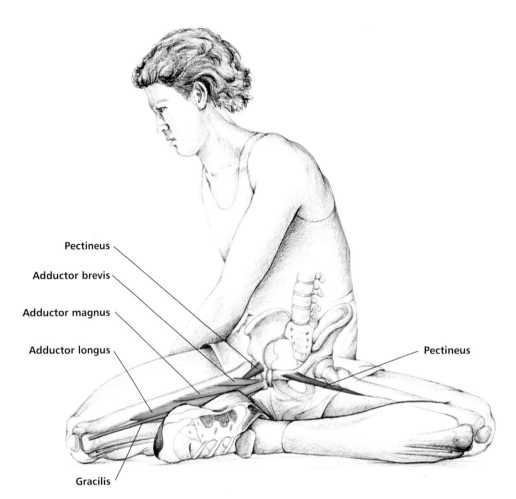

Pectineus

Adductor brevis

Adductor magnus

Adductor longus

Pectineus

Gracilis

Technique
Sit with one leg crossed and your other leg behind your buttocks. Lean your whole body towards the leg that is behind your buttocks.

Muscles being stretched
Primary muscle: Pectineus.
Secondary muscles: Adductor longus, brevis and magnus. Gracilis.

Sports that benefit from this stretch
Cycling. Hiking. Backpacking. Mountaineering. Orienteering. Ice hockey. Field hockey. Ice-skating. Roller-skating. Inline skating. Martial arts. Running. Track. Cross-country. American football (gridiron). Soccer. Rugby. Snow skiing. Water skiing. Walking. Race walking.

Sports injury where stretch may be useful
Groin strain. Tendonitis of the adductor muscles. Snapping hip syndrome. Trochanteric bursitis.

Additional information for performing this stretch correctly
The more you lean your whole body towards the leg that is behind your buttocks, the more tension you will feel.

Complementary stretch
056.

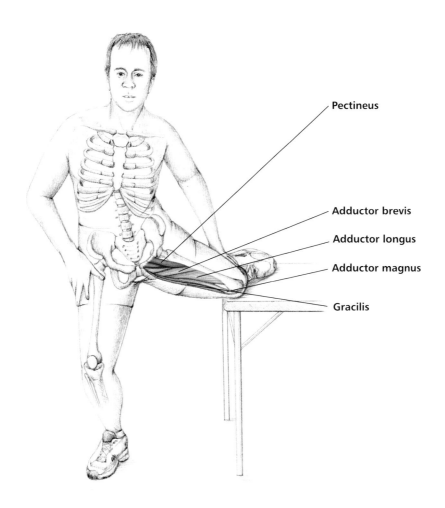

Pectineus

Adductor brevis

Adductor longus

Adductor magnus

Gracilis

Technique
Stand beside a table and raise your lower leg out to the side and up onto the table. Then slowly lower your body.

Muscles being stretched
Primary muscle: Pectineus.
Secondary muscles: Adductor longus, brevis and magnus. Gracilis.

Sports that benefit from this stretch
Cycling. Hiking. Backpacking. Mountaineering. Orienteering. Ice hockey. Field hockey. Ice-skating. Roller-skating. Inline skating. Martial arts. Running. Track. Cross-country. American football (gridiron). Soccer. Rugby. Snow skiing. Water skiing. Walking. Race walking.

Sports injury where stretch may be useful
Groin strain. Tendonitis of the adductor muscles. Snapping hip syndrome. Trochanteric bursitis.

Common problems and additional information for performing this stretch correctly
Use the leg you are standing on to regulate the intensity of this stretch. The lower you go, the more tension you will feel.

Complementary stretch
055.

057: SITTING CROSS-LEGGED REACH FORWARD STRETCH

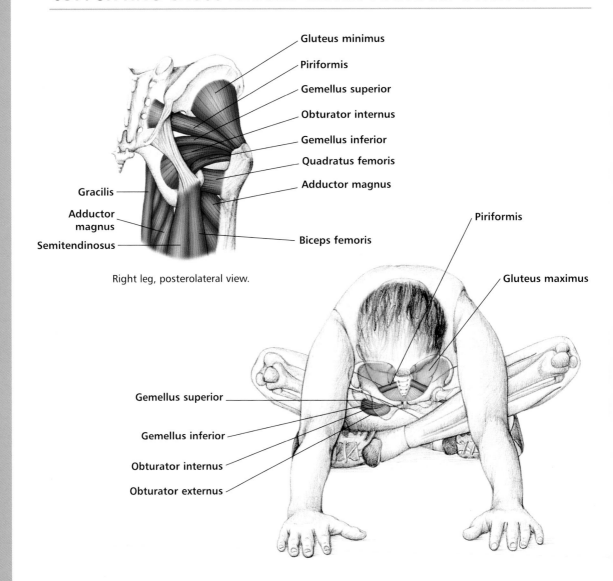

Gluteus minimus

Piriformis

Gemellus superior

Obturator internus

Gemellus inferior

Quadratus femoris

Adductor magnus

Gracilis

Adductor magnus

Semitendinosus

Biceps femoris

Right leg, posterolateral view.

Piriformis

Gluteus maximus

Gemellus superior

Gemellus inferior

Obturator internus

Obturator externus

Technique
Sit cross-legged and keep your back straight. Then gently lean forward.

Muscles being stretched
Primary muscles: Piriformis. Gemellus superior and inferior. Obturator internus and externus. Quadratus femoris.
Secondary muscle: Gluteus maximus.

Sports that benefit from this stretch
Cycling. Hiking. Backpacking. Mountaineering. Orienteering. Ice hockey. Field hockey. Ice-skating. Roller-skating. Inline skating. Martial arts. Rowing. Canoeing. Kayaking. Running. Track. Cross-country. American football (gridiron). Soccer. Rugby. Snow skiing. Water skiing. Walking. Race walking.

Sports injury where stretch may be useful
Piriformis syndrome. Groin strain. Tendonitis of the adductor muscles. Snapping hip syndrome. Trochanteric bursitis.

Common problems and additional information for performing this stretch correctly
Make the emphasis of this stretch keeping your back straight, rather than trying to lean too far forward.

Complementary stretch
058.

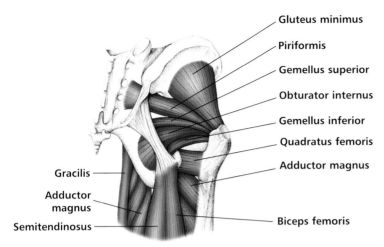

Gluteus minimus
Piriformis
Gemellus superior
Obturator internus
Gemellus inferior
Quadratus femoris
Adductor magnus

Gracilis
Adductor magnus
Semitendinosus

Biceps femoris

Right leg, posterolateral view.

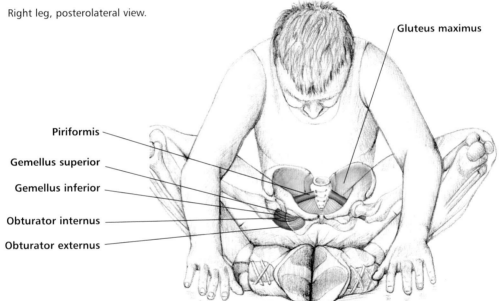

Gluteus maximus

Piriformis
Gemellus superior
Gemellus inferior
Obturator internus
Obturator externus

Technique
Sit with the soles of your feet together and keep your back straight. Then gently lean forward.

Muscles being stretched
Primary muscles: Piriformis. Gemellus superior and inferior. Obturator internus and externus. Quadratus femoris.
Secondary muscle: Gluteus maximus.

Sports that benefit from this stretch
Cycling. Hiking. Backpacking. Mountaineering. Orienteering. Ice hockey. Field hockey. Ice-skating. Roller-skating. Inline skating. Martial arts. Rowing. Canoeing. Kayaking. Running. Track. Cross-country. American football (gridiron). Soccer. Rugby. Snow skiing. Water skiing. Walking. Race walking.

Sports injury where stretch may be useful
Piriformis syndrome. Groin strain. Tendonitis of the adductor muscles. Snapping hip syndrome. Trochanteric bursitis.

Common problems and additional information for performing this stretch correctly
Make the emphasis of this stretch keeping your back straight, rather than trying to lean too far forward.

Complementary stretch
057.

059: SITTING KNEE-TO-CHEST BUTTOCKS STRETCH

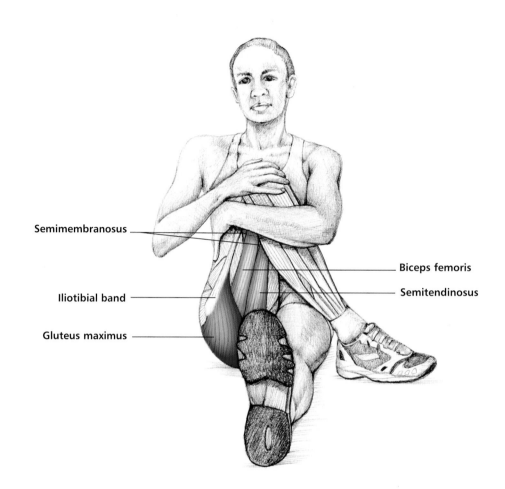

Semimembranosus

Biceps femoris

Iliotibial band

Semitendinosus

Gluteus maximus

Technique
Sit with one leg straight and the other leg crossed over your knee. Pull the raised knee towards your opposite shoulder while keeping your back straight and your shoulders facing forward.

Muscles being stretched
Primary muscle: Gluteus maximus.
Secondary muscles: Semimembranosus. Semitendinosus. Biceps femoris.

Sports that benefit from this stretch
Cycling. Hiking. Backpacking. Mountaineering. Orienteering. Ice hockey. Field hockey. Ice-skating. Roller-skating. Inline skating. Martial arts. Running. Track. Cross-country. American football (gridiron). Soccer. Rugby. Snow skiing. Water skiing. Walking. Race walking.

Sports injury where stretch may be useful
Lower back muscle strain. Lower back ligament sprain. Hamstring strain. Iliotibial band syndrome.

Common problems and additional information for performing this stretch correctly
Keeping your back straight and your shoulders facing forward will ensure that your buttocks get the maximum benefit from this stretch. Resist the temptation to rotate your shoulders towards your knee.

Complementary stretch
051.

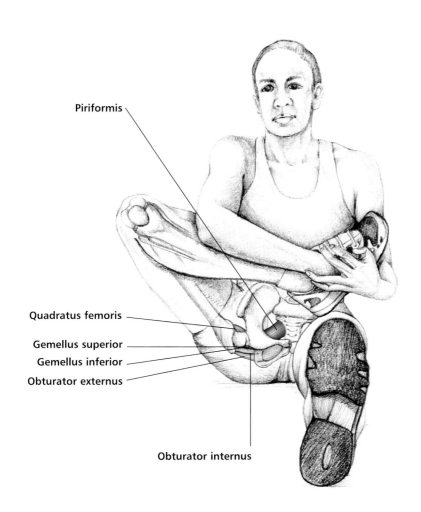

Piriformis

Quadratus femoris

Gemellus superior

Gemellus inferior

Obturator externus

Obturator internus

Technique
Sit with one leg straight and hold onto your other ankle. Pull it directly towards your chest.

Muscles being stretched
Primary muscle: Piriformis.
Secondary muscles: Gemellus superior and inferior. Obturator internus and externus. Quadratus femoris.

Sports that benefit from this stretch
Cycling. Hiking. Backpacking. Mountaineering. Orienteering. Ice hockey. Field hockey. Ice-skating. Roller-skating. Inline skating. Martial arts. Running. Track. Cross-country. American football (gridiron). Soccer. Rugby. Snow skiing. Water skiing. Walking. Race walking.

Sports injury where stretch may be useful
Piriformis syndrome. Snapping hip syndrome. Trochanteric bursitis.

Common problems and additional information for performing this stretch correctly
Use your hands and arms to regulate the intensity of this stretch. The closer you pull your foot to your chest, the more intense the stretch.

Complementary stretch
054.

061: LYING CROSS-OVER KNEE PULL-UP STRETCH

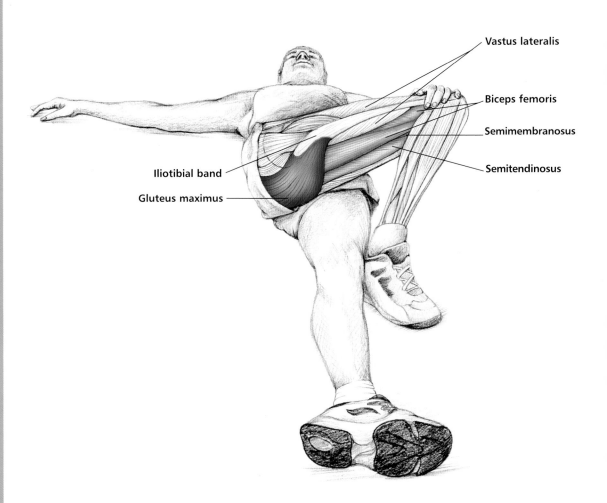

Vastus lateralis

Biceps femoris

Semimembranosus

Semitendinosus

Iliotibial band

Gluteus maximus

Technique
Lie on your back and cross one leg over the other. Bring your foot up to your opposite knee and with your opposite arm pull your raised knee up towards your chest.

Muscles being stretched
Primary muscle: Gluteus maximus.
Secondary muscles: Semimembranosus. Semitendinosus. Biceps femoris.

Sports that benefit from this stretch
Cycling. Hiking. Backpacking. Mountaineering. Orienteering. Ice hockey. Field hockey. Ice-skating. Roller-skating. Inline skating. Martial arts. Running. Track. Cross-country. American football (gridiron). Soccer. Rugby. Snow skiing. Water skiing. Walking. Race walking.

Sports injury where stretch may be useful
Lower back muscle strain. Lower back ligament sprain. Hamstring strain. Iliotibial band syndrome.

Additional information for performing this stretch correctly
Keep your shoulders on the ground and concentrate on pulling your raised knee up towards your chest, not down towards the ground.

Complementary stretch
059.

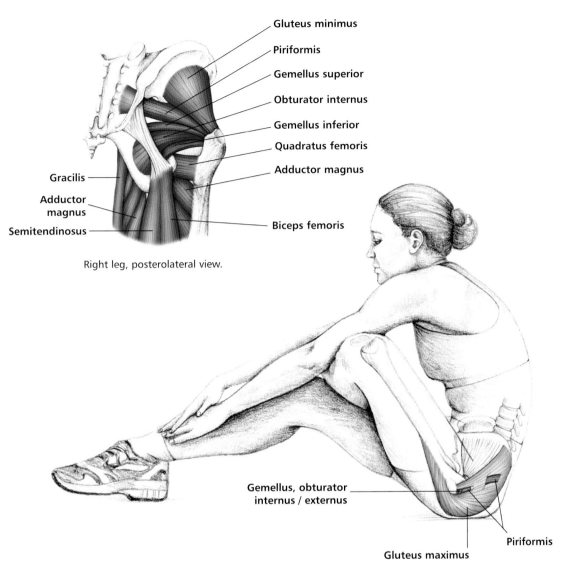

Gluteus minimus
Piriformis
Gemellus superior
Obturator internus
Gemellus inferior
Quadratus femoris
Adductor magnus
Gracilis
Adductor magnus
Semitendinosus
Biceps femoris

Right leg, posterolateral view.

Gemellus, obturator internus / externus
Piriformis
Gluteus maximus

Technique
Sit with one leg slightly bent. Raise the other foot up onto your raised leg and rest it on your thigh, then slowly lean forward.

Muscles being stretched
Primary muscles: Piriformis. Gemellus superior and inferior. Obturator internus and externus. Quadratus femoris.
Secondary muscle: Gluteus maximus.

Sports that benefit from this stretch
Cycling. Hiking. Backpacking. Mountaineering. Orienteering. Ice hockey. Field hockey. Ice-skating. Roller-skating. Inline skating. Martial arts. Running. Track. Cross-country. American football (gridiron). Soccer. Rugby. Snow skiing. Water skiing. Walking. Race walking.

Sports injury where stretch may be useful
Piriformis syndrome. Snapping hip syndrome. Trochanteric bursitis.

Common problems and additional information for performing this stretch correctly
This position can be a little hard to get into, so make sure that you are well supported and use your hands for balance if you need to. To increase the intensity of this stretch, straighten your back and lean forward.

Complementary stretch
060.

063: LYING LEG RESTING BUTTOCKS STRETCH

STRETCHES FOR THE HIPS AND BUTTOCKS

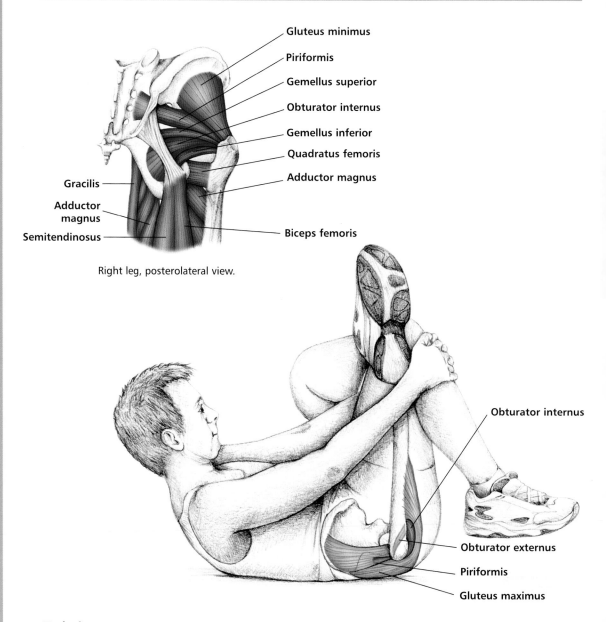

Right leg, posterolateral view.

Technique
Lie on your back and slightly bend one leg. Raise the other foot up onto your bent leg and rest it on your thigh. Then reach forward, holding onto your knee and pull towards you.

Muscles being stretched
Primary muscles: Piriformis. Gemellus superior and inferior. Obturator internus and externus. Quadratus femoris.
Secondary muscle: Gluteus maximus.

Sports that benefit from this stretch
Cycling. Hiking. Backpacking. Mountaineering. Orienteering. Ice hockey. Field hockey. Ice-skating. Roller-skating. Inline skating. Martial arts. Running. Track. Cross-country. American football (gridiron). Soccer. Rugby. Snow skiing. Water skiing. Walking. Race walking.

Sports injury where stretch may be useful
Piriformis syndrome. Snapping hip syndrome. Trochanteric bursitis.

Additional information for performing this stretch correctly
Regulate the intensity of this stretch by pulling your knee towards you.

Complementary stretch
062.

11 Stretches for the Quadriceps

064: KNEELING QUAD STRETCH

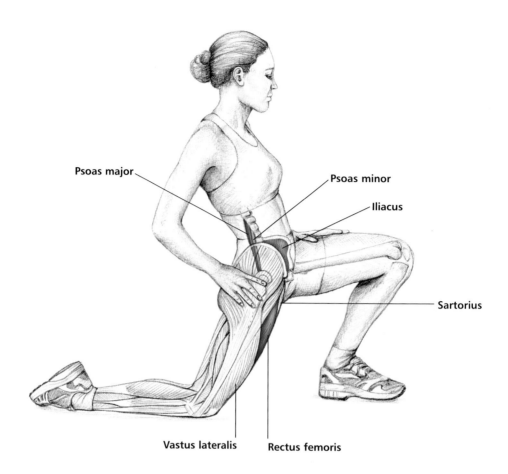

Psoas major

Psoas minor

Iliacus

Sartorius

Vastus lateralis

Rectus femoris

Technique
Kneel on one foot and the other knee. If needed, hold on to something to keep your balance. Push your hips forward.

Muscles being stretched
Primary muscles: Iliacus. Psoas major. Rectus femoris.
Secondary muscle: Psoas minor.

Sports that benefit from this stretch
Cycling. Hiking. Backpacking. Mountaineering. Orienteering. Ice hockey. Field hockey. Ice-skating. Roller-skating. Inline skating. Martial arts. Running. Track. Cross-country. American football (gridiron). Soccer. Rugby. Snow skiing. Water skiing. Surfing. Walking. Race walking.

Sports injury where stretch may be useful
Hip flexor strain. Avulsion fracture in the pelvic area. Osteitis pubis. Iliopsoas tendonitis. Trochanteric bursitis. Quadriceps strain. Quadriceps tendonitis.

Common problems and additional information for performing this stretch correctly
Regulate the intensity of this stretch by pushing your hips forward. If need be, place a towel or mat under your knee for comfort.

Complementary stretch
067.

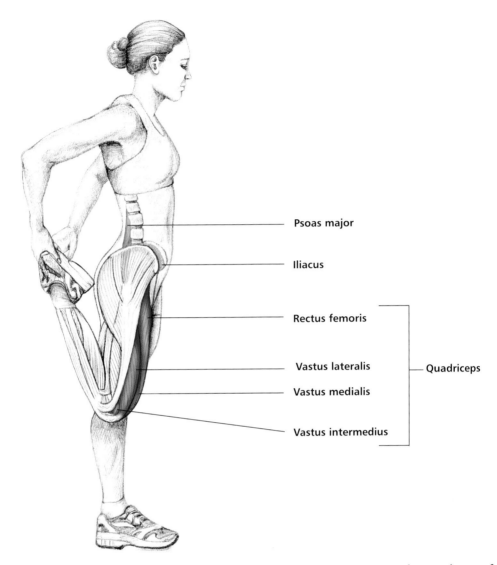

Psoas major

Iliacus

Rectus femoris

Vastus lateralis — Quadriceps

Vastus medialis

Vastus intermedius

Technique
Stand upright while balancing on one leg. Pull your other foot up behind your buttocks and keep your knees together while pushing your hips forward. Hold on to something for balance.

Muscles being stretched
Primary muscles: Rectus femoris. Vastus medialis, lateralis and intermedius.
Secondary muscles: Iliacus. Psoas major.

Sports that benefit from this stretch
Cycling. Hiking. Backpacking. Mountaineering. Orienteering. Ice hockey. Field hockey. Ice-skating. Roller-skating. Inline skating. Martial arts. Running. Track. Cross-country. American football (gridiron). Soccer. Rugby. Snow skiing. Water skiing. Surfing. Walking. Race walking.

Sports injury where stretch may be useful
Hip flexor strain. Avulsion fracture in the pelvic area. Osteitis pubis. Iliopsoas tendonitis. Trochanteric bursitis. Quadriceps strain. Quadriceps tendonitis. Patellofemoral pain syndrome. Patellar tendonitis. Subluxing kneecap.

Common problems and additional information for performing this stretch correctly
This position can put undue pressure on the knee joint and ligaments. Anyone with knee pain or knee injury should avoid this stretch.

Complementary stretch
066.

066: LYING QUAD STRETCH

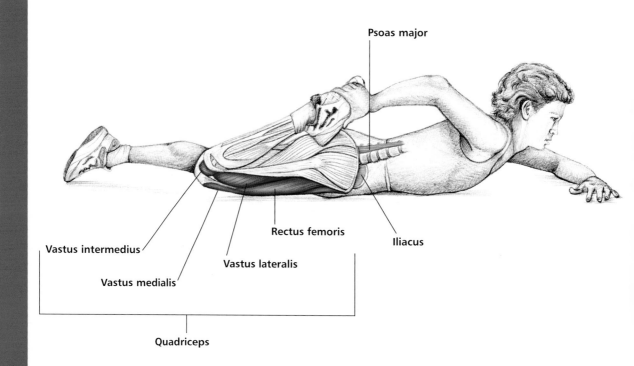

Psoas major

Rectus femoris

Iliacus

Vastus intermedius

Vastus lateralis

Vastus medialis

Quadriceps

Technique
Lie face down and pull one foot up behind your buttocks.

Muscles being stretched
Primary muscles: Rectus femoris. Vastus medialis, lateralis and intermedius.
Secondary muscles: Iliacus. Psoas major.

Sports that benefit from this stretch
Cycling. Hiking. Backpacking. Mountaineering. Orienteering. Ice hockey. Field hockey. Ice-skating. Roller-skating. Inline skating. Martial arts. Running. Track. Cross-country. American football (gridiron). Soccer. Rugby. Snow skiing. Water skiing. Surfing. Walking. Race walking.

Sports injury where stretch may be useful
Hip flexor strain. Avulsion fracture in the pelvic area. Osteitis pubis. Iliopsoas tendonitis. Trochanteric bursitis. Quadriceps strain. Quadriceps tendonitis. Patellofemoral pain syndrome. Patellar tendonitis. Subluxing kneecap.

Common problems and additional information for performing this stretch correctly
This position can put undue pressure on the knee joint and ligaments. Anyone with knee pain or knee injury should avoid this stretch.

Complementary stretch
065.

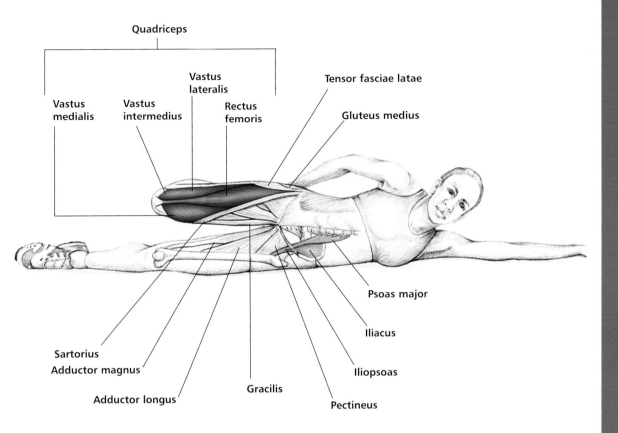

Quadriceps

Vastus lateralis

Tensor fasciae latae

Vastus medialis

Vastus intermedius

Rectus femoris

Gluteus medius

Psoas major

Iliacus

Sartorius
Adductor magnus

Iliopsoas

Adductor longus

Gracilis

Pectineus

Technique
Lie on your side and pull your top leg behind your buttocks. Keep your knees together and push your hips forward.

Muscles being stretched
Primary muscles: Rectus femoris. Vastus medialis, lateralis and intermedius.
Secondary muscles: Iliacus. Psoas major.

Sports that benefit from this stretch
Cycling. Hiking. Backpacking. Mountaineering. Orienteering. Ice hockey. Field hockey. Ice-skating. Roller-skating. Inline skating. Martial arts. Running. Track. Cross-country. American football (gridiron). Soccer. Rugby. Snow skiing. Water skiing. Surfing. Walking. Race walking.

Sports injury where stretch may be useful
Hip flexor strain. Avulsion fracture in the pelvic area. Osteitis pubis. Iliopsoas tendonitis. Trochanteric bursitis. Quadriceps strain. Quadriceps tendonitis. Patellofemoral pain syndrome. Patellar tendonitis. Subluxing kneecap.

Common problems and additional information for performing this stretch correctly
This position can put undue pressure on the knee joint and ligaments. Anyone with knee pain or knee injury should avoid this stretch.

Complementary stretch
064.

068: DOUBLE LEAN-BACK QUAD STRETCH

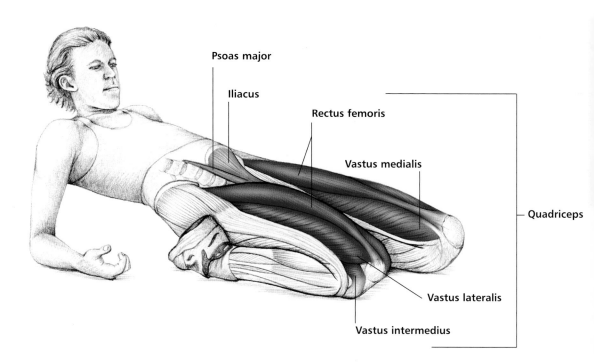

Psoas major

Iliacus

Rectus femoris

Vastus medialis

Quadriceps

Vastus lateralis

Vastus intermedius

Technique

Sit on the ground and bend one or both knees and place your legs under your buttocks. Then slowly lean backwards.

Muscles being stretched

Primary muscles: Rectus femoris. Vastus medialis, lateralis and intermedius.
Secondary muscles: Iliacus. Psoas major.

Sports that benefit from this stretch

Cycling. Hiking. Backpacking. Mountaineering. Orienteering. Ice hockey. Field hockey. Ice-skating. Roller-skating. Inline skating. Martial arts. Running. Track. Cross-country. American football (gridiron). Soccer. Rugby. Snow skiing. Water skiing. Surfing. Walking. Race walking.

Sports injury where stretch may be useful

Hip flexor strain. Avulsion fracture in the pelvic area. Osteitis pubis. Iliopsoas tendonitis. Trochanteric bursitis. Quadriceps strain. Quadriceps tendonitis. Patellofemoral pain syndrome. Patellar tendonitis. Subluxing kneecap.

Common problems and additional information for performing this stretch correctly

This position can put undue pressure on the knee joint and ligaments. Anyone with knee pain or knee injury should avoid this stretch.

Complementary stretch

065.

12 Stretches for the Hamstrings

069: SITTING REACH FORWARD HAMSTRING STRETCH

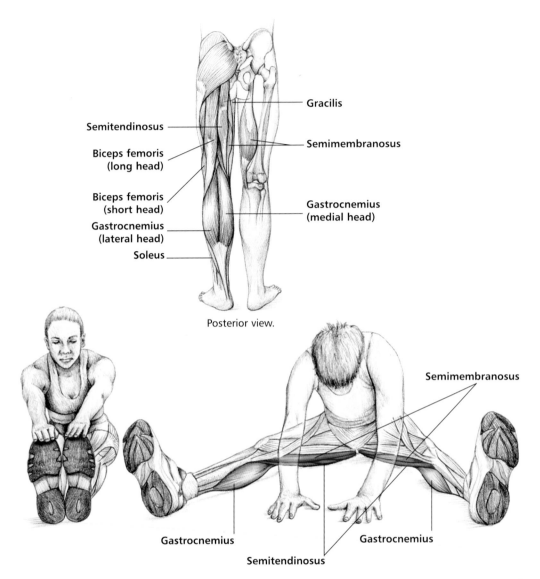

Posterior view.

Technique
Sit with both legs straight out in front and keep your toes pointing straight up. Make sure your back is straight and then reach forward towards your toes.

Muscles being stretched
Primary muscles: Semimembranosus. Semitendinosus. Biceps femoris.
Secondary muscle: Gastrocnemius.

Sports that benefit from this stretch
Basketball. Netball. Cycling. Hiking. Backpacking. Mountaineering. Orienteering. Ice hockey. Field hockey. Ice-skating. Roller-skating. Inline skating. Martial arts. Running. Track. Cross-country. American football (gridiron). Soccer. Rugby. Snow skiing. Water skiing. Surfing. Walking. Race walking. Wrestling.

Sports injury where stretch may be useful
Lower back muscle strain. Lower back ligament sprain. Hamstring strain.

Common problems and additional information for performing this stretch correctly
It is important to keep your toes pointing straight upwards. Letting your toes fall to one side will cause this stretch to put uneven tension on the hamstring muscles. Over an extended period of time, this could lead to a muscle imbalance.

Complementary stretch
073.

070: STANDING TOE-POINTED HAMSTRING STRETCH

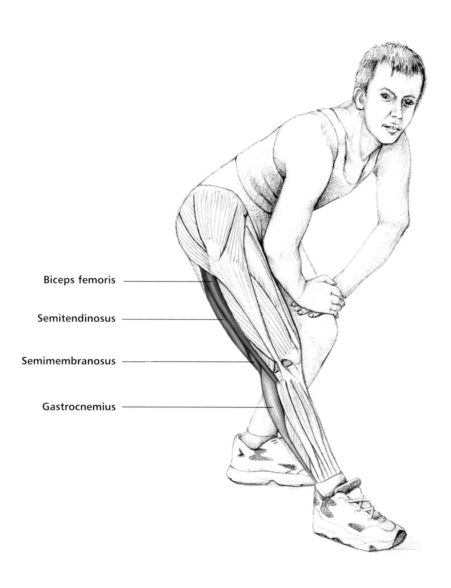

Biceps femoris

Semitendinosus

Semimembranosus

Gastrocnemius

Technique
Stand with one knee bent and the other leg straight out in front. Point your toes towards the ground and lean forward. Keep your back straight and rest your hands on your bent knee.

Muscles being stretched
Primary muscles: Semimembranosus. Semi-tendinosus. Biceps femoris.
Secondary muscle: Gastrocnemius.

Sports that benefit from this stretch
Basketball. Netball. Cycling. Hiking. Backpacking. Mountaineering. Orienteering. Ice hockey. Field hockey. Ice-skating. Roller-skating. Inline skating. Martial arts. Running. Track. Cross-country. American football (gridiron). Soccer. Rugby. Snow skiing. Water skiing. Surfing. Walking. Race walking. Wrestling.

Sports injury where stretch may be useful
Lower back muscle strain. Lower back ligament sprain. Hamstring strain.

Additional information for performing this stretch correctly
Regulate the intensity of this stretch by keeping your back straight and leaning forward.

Complementary stretch
071.

071: STANDING TOE-RAISED HAMSTRING STRETCH

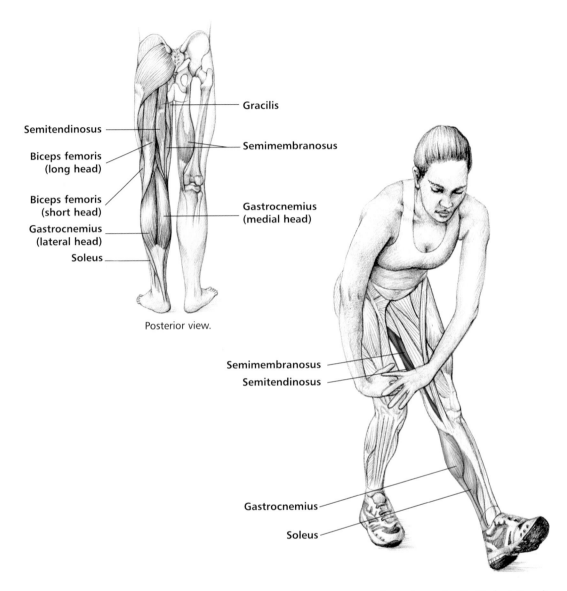

Posterior view.

Technique

Stand with one knee bent and the other leg straight out in front. Point your toes towards your body and lean forward. Keep your back straight and rest your hands on your bent knee.

Muscles being stretched

Primary muscles: Semimembranosus. Semitendinosus. Biceps femoris.
Secondary muscles: Gastrocnemius. Soleus.

Sports that benefit from this stretch

Basketball. Netball. Cycling. Hiking. Backpacking. Mountaineering. Orienteering. Ice hockey. Field hockey. Ice-skating. Roller-skating. Inline skating. Martial arts. Running. Track. Cross-country. American football (gridiron). Soccer. Rugby. Snow skiing. Water skiing. Surfing. Walking. Race walking. Wrestling.

Sports injury where stretch may be useful

Lower back muscle strain. Lower back ligament sprain. Hamstring strain. Calf strain.

Additional information for performing this stretch correctly

Regulate the intensity of this stretch by keeping your back straight and flexing your ankle so that your toes are pointing upwards.

Complementary stretch

072.

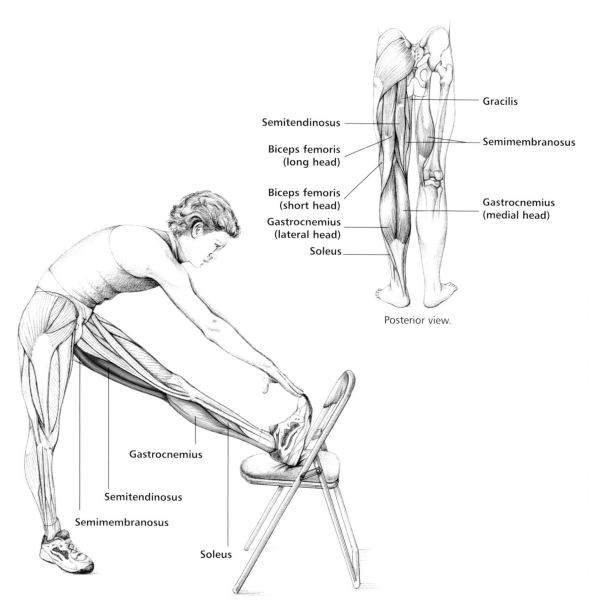

Posterior view.

Technique
Stand upright and raise one leg on to an object. Keep that leg straight and your toes pointing straight up. Lean forward while keeping your back straight.

Muscles being stretched
Primary muscles: Semimembranosus. Semitendinosus. Biceps femoris.
Secondary muscles: Gastrocnemius. Soleus.

Sports that benefit from this stretch
Basketball. Netball. Cycling. Hiking. Backpacking. Mountaineering. Orienteering. Ice hockey. Field hockey. Ice-skating. Roller-skating. Inline skating. Martial arts. Running. Track. Cross-country. American football (gridiron). Soccer. Rugby. Snow skiing. Water skiing. Surfing. Walking. Race walking. Wrestling.

Sports injury where stretch may be useful
Lower back muscle strain. Lower back ligament sprain. Hamstring strain. Calf strain.

Common problems and additional information for performing this stretch correctly
Regulate the intensity of this stretch by keeping your back straight and leaning forward.

Complementary stretch
069.

073: SITTING SINGLE LEG HAMSTRING STRETCH

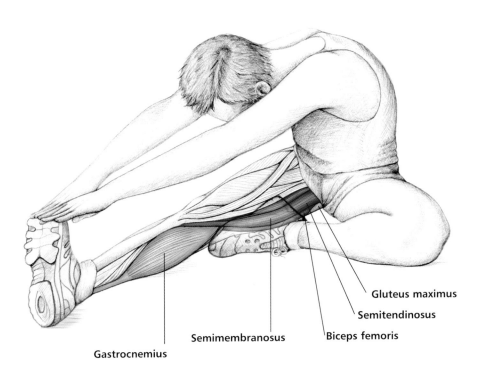

Gluteus maximus

Semitendinosus

Biceps femoris

Semimembranosus

Gastrocnemius

Technique
Sit with one leg straight out in front and toes pointing upwards. Bring your other foot towards your knee. Let your head fall forward and reach towards your toes with both hands.

Muscles being stretched
Primary muscles: Semimembranosus. Semitendinosus. Biceps femoris.
Secondary muscles: Gastrocnemius. Gluteus maximus.

Sports that benefit from this stretch
Basketball. Netball. Cycling. Hiking. Backpacking. Mountaineering. Orienteering. Ice hockey. Field hockey. Ice-skating. Roller-skating. Inline skating. Martial arts. Running. Track. Cross-country. American football (gridiron). Soccer. Rugby. Snow skiing. Water skiing. Surfing. Walking. Race walking. Wrestling.

Sports injury where stretch may be useful
Lower back muscle strain. Lower back ligament sprain. Hamstring strain. Calf strain.

Common problems and additional information for performing this stretch correctly
It is important to keep your toes pointing straight upwards. Letting your toes fall to one side will cause this stretch to put uneven tension on the hamstring muscles. Over an extended period of time, this could lead to a muscle imbalance.

Complementary stretch
076.

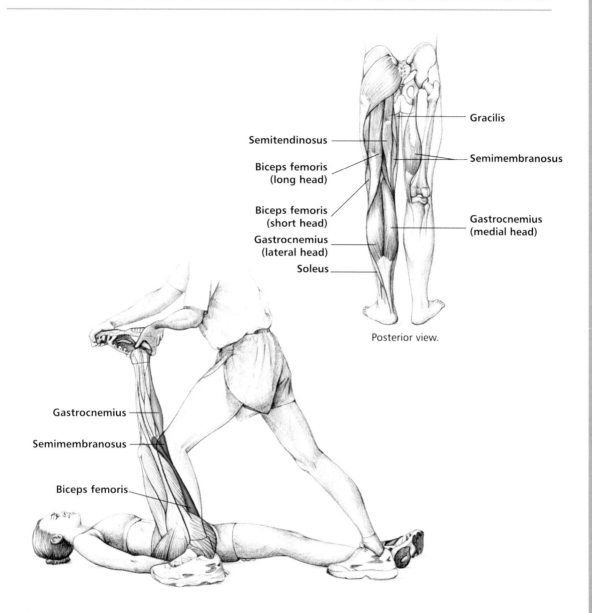

Posterior view.

Technique
Lie on your back and keep both legs straight. Have a partner raise one of your legs off the ground and as far back as is comfortable. Make sure your toes are pointing directly backwards.

Muscles being stretched
Primary muscles: Semimembranosus. Semitendinosus. Biceps femoris.
Secondary muscle: Gastrocnemius.

Sports that benefit from this stretch
Basketball. Netball. Cycling. Hiking. Backpacking. Mountaineering. Orienteering. Ice hockey. Field hockey. Ice-skating. Roller-skating. Inline skating. Martial arts. Running. Track. Cross-country. American football (gridiron). Soccer. Rugby. Snow skiing. Water skiing. Surfing. Walking. Race walking. Wrestling.

Sports injury where stretch may be useful
Lower back muscle strain. Lower back ligament sprain. Hamstring strain. Calf strain.

Common problems and additional information for performing this stretch correctly
Choose your stretching partner carefully. They are responsible for your safety while performing this stretch, so make sure you communicate clearly with them at all times.

Complementary stretch
072.

075: LYING BENT KNEE HAMSTRING STRETCH

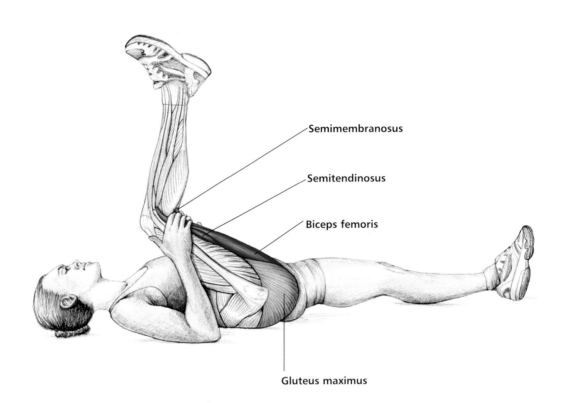

Semimembranosus

Semitendinosus

Biceps femoris

Gluteus maximus

Technique
Lie on your back and bend one leg. Pull the other knee towards your chest, then slowly and gently straighten your raised leg.

Muscles being stretched
Primary muscles: Semimembranosus. Semitendinosus. Biceps femoris.
Secondary muscle: Gluteus maximus.

Sports that benefit from this stretch
Basketball. Netball. Cycling. Hiking. Backpacking. Mountaineering. Orienteering. Ice hockey. Field hockey. Ice-skating. Roller-skating. Inline skating. Martial arts. Running. Track. Cross-country. American football (gridiron). Soccer. Rugby. Snow skiing. Water skiing. Surfing. Walking. Race walking. Wrestling.

Sports injury where stretch may be useful
Lower back muscle strain. Lower back ligament sprain. Hamstring strain.

Additional information for performing this stretch correctly
Keep your upper leg (thigh) relatively still, and regulate the intensity of this stretch by straightening your knee.

Complementary stretch
079.

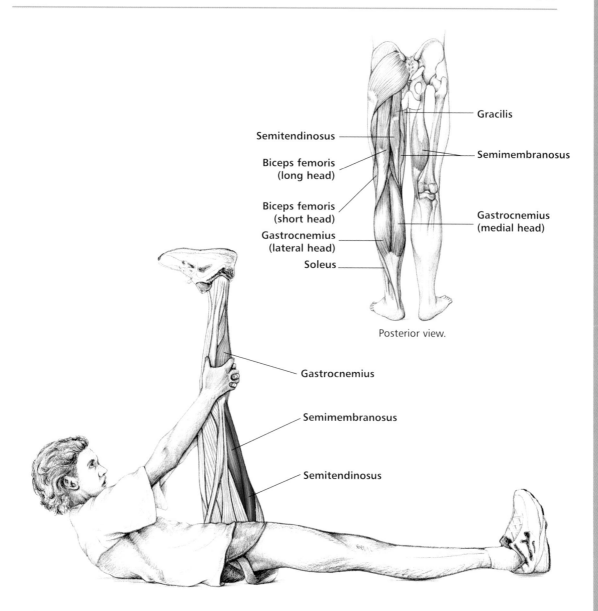

Gracilis

Semitendinosus

Biceps femoris
(long head)

Semimembranosus

Biceps femoris
(short head)

Gastrocnemius
(medial head)

Gastrocnemius
(lateral head)

Soleus

Posterior view.

Gastrocnemius

Semimembranosus

Semitendinosus

Technique
Lie on your back and bend one leg. Raise your straight leg and pull it towards your chest.

Muscles being stretched
Primary muscles: Semimembranosus. Semi-tendinosus. Biceps femoris.
Secondary muscle: Gastrocnemius.

Sports that benefit from this stretch
Basketball. Netball. Cycling. Hiking. Backpacking. Mountaineering. Orienteering. Ice hockey. Field hockey. Ice-skating. Roller-skating. Inline skating. Martial arts. Running. Track. Cross-country. American football (gridiron). Soccer. Rugby. Snow skiing. Water skiing. Surfing. Walking. Race walking. Wrestling.

Sports injury where stretch may be useful
Lower back muscle strain. Lower back ligament sprain. Hamstring strain. Calf strain.

Common problems and additional information for performing this stretch correctly
It is important to keep your toes pointing straight backwards. Letting your toes fall to one side will cause this stretch to put uneven tension on the hamstring muscles. Over an extended period of time, this could lead to a muscle imbalance.

Complementary stretch
077.

077: KNEELING TOE-RAISED HAMSTRING STRETCH

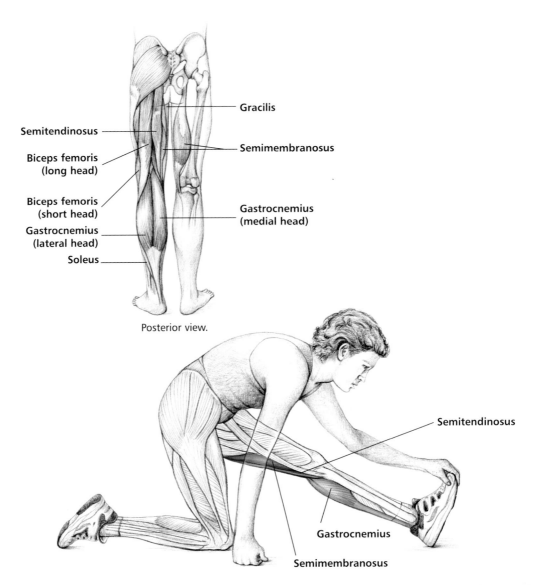

Posterior view.

Technique
Kneel on one knee and place your other leg forward with your heel on the ground. Keep your back straight and point your toes towards your body. Reach towards your toes with one hand.

Muscles being stretched
Primary muscles: Semimembranosus. Semitendinosus. Biceps femoris.
Secondary muscle: Gastrocnemius.

Sports that benefit from this stretch
Basketball. Netball. Cycling. Hiking. Backpacking. Mountaineering. Orienteering. Ice hockey. Field hockey. Ice-skating. Roller-skating. Inline skating. Martial arts. Running. Track. Cross-country. American football (gridiron). Soccer. Rugby. Snow skiing. Water skiing. Surfing. Walking. Race walking. Wrestling.

Sports injury where stretch may be useful
Lower back muscle strain. Lower back ligament sprain. Hamstring strain. Calf strain.

Common problems and additional information for performing this stretch correctly
It is not important to be able to touch your toes. Concentrate on keeping your back straight and your toes pointing up.

Complementary stretch
071.

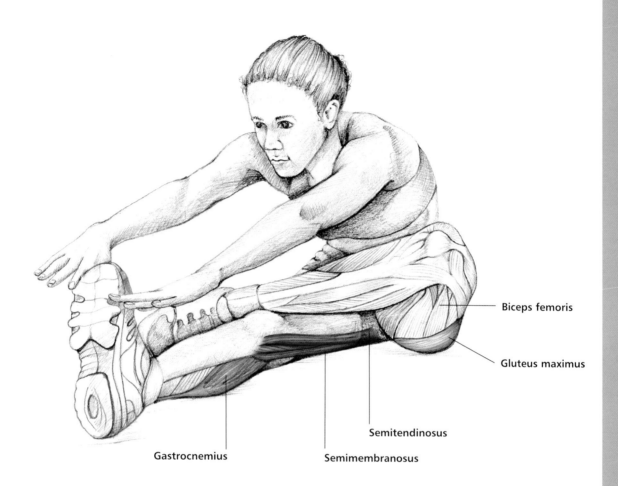

Biceps femoris

Gluteus maximus

Semitendinosus

Semimembranosus

Gastrocnemius

Technique
Sit with one leg straight out in front and keep your toes pointing up. Cross your other leg over and rest your foot on your thigh. Lean forward, keep your back straight and reach for your toes.

Muscles being stretched
Primary muscles: Semimembranosus. Semitendinosus. Biceps femoris.
Secondary muscles: Gastrocnemius. Gluteus maximus.

Sports that benefit from this stretch
Basketball. Netball. Cycling. Hiking. Backpacking. Mountaineering. Orienteering. Ice hockey. Field hockey. Ice-skating. Roller-skating. Inline skating. Martial arts. Running. Track. Cross-country. American football (gridiron). Soccer. Rugby. Snow skiing. Water skiing. Surfing. Walking. Race walking. Wrestling.

Sports injury where stretch may be useful
Lower back muscle strain. Lower back ligament sprain. Hamstring strain. Calf strain.

Additional information for performing this stretch correctly
It is not important to be able to touch your toes. Simply reaching towards your toes is sufficient.

Complementary stretch
074.

079: STANDING LEG-UP BENT KNEE HAMSTRING STRETCH

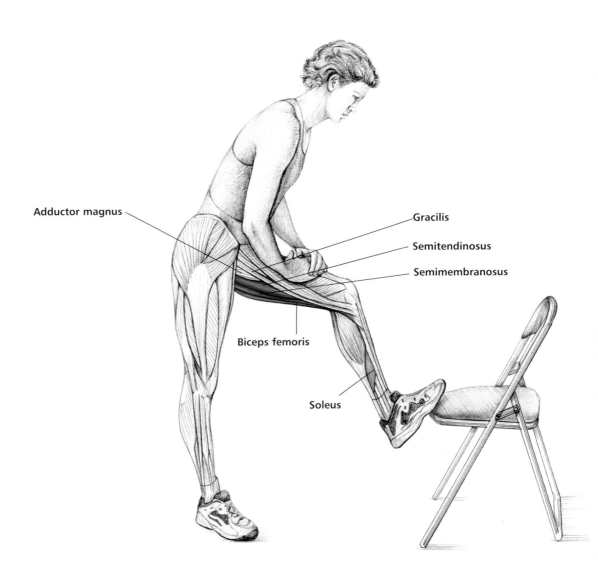

Adductor magnus

Gracilis

Semitendinosus

Semimembranosus

Biceps femoris

Soleus

Technique
Stand with one foot raised onto a chair or an object. Keep your leg slightly bent and let your heel drop off the edge of the object. Keep your back straight and move your chest towards your thigh.

Muscles being stretched
Primary muscles: Semimembranosus. Semitendinosus. Biceps femoris.
Secondary muscle: Soleus.

Sports that benefit from this stretch
Basketball. Netball. Cycling. Hiking. Backpacking. Mountaineering. Orienteering. Ice hockey. Field hockey. Ice-skating. Roller-skating. Inline skating. Martial arts. Running. Track. Cross-country. American football (gridiron). Soccer. Rugby. Snow skiing. Water skiing. Surfing. Walking. Race walking. Wrestling.

Sports injury where stretch may be useful
Hamstring strain. Achilles tendon strain. Achilles tendonitis. Medial tibial pain syndrome (shin splints).

Additional information for performing this stretch correctly
Pushing your heel down towards the ground will help to intensify this stretch.

Complementary stretch
080.

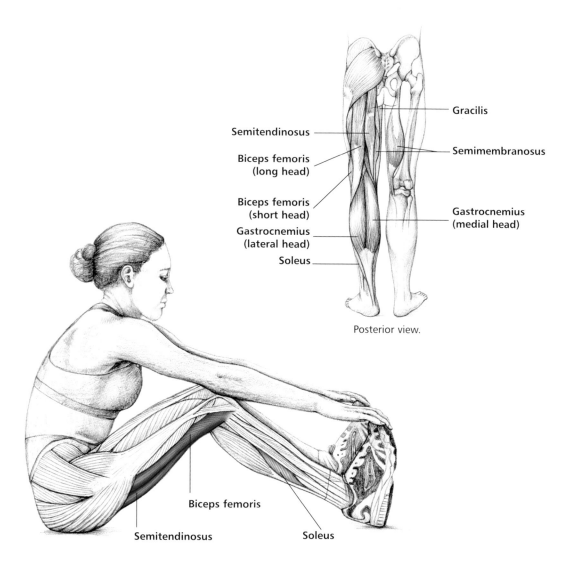

Gracilis

Semitendinosus

Semimembranosus

Biceps femoris
(long head)

Biceps femoris
(short head)

Gastrocnemius
(medial head)

Gastrocnemius
(lateral head)

Soleus

Posterior view.

Biceps femoris

Semitendinosus

Soleus

Technique
Sit on the ground with your legs slightly bent. Hold onto your toes with your hands and pull your toes towards your body. Lean forward and keep your back straight.

Muscles being stretched
Primary muscles: Semimembranosus. Semitendinosus. Biceps femoris.
Secondary muscle: Soleus.

Sports that benefit from this stretch
Basketball. Netball. Cycling. Hiking. Backpacking. Mountaineering. Orienteering. Ice hockey. Field hockey. Ice-skating. Roller-skating. Inline skating. Martial arts. Running. Track. Cross-country. American football (gridiron). Soccer. Rugby. Snow skiing. Water skiing. Surfing. Walking. Race walking. Wrestling.

Sports injury where stretch may be useful
Hamstring strain. Achilles tendon strain. Achilles tendonitis. Medial tibial pain syndrome (shin splints).

Common problems and additional information for performing this stretch correctly
When pulling back on your toes, make sure they are pointing straight upwards. Letting your toes fall to one side will cause this stretch to put uneven tension on the hamstring muscles. Over an extended period of time, this could lead to a muscle imbalance.

Complementary stretch
075.

081: STANDING REACH DOWN HAMSTRING STRETCH

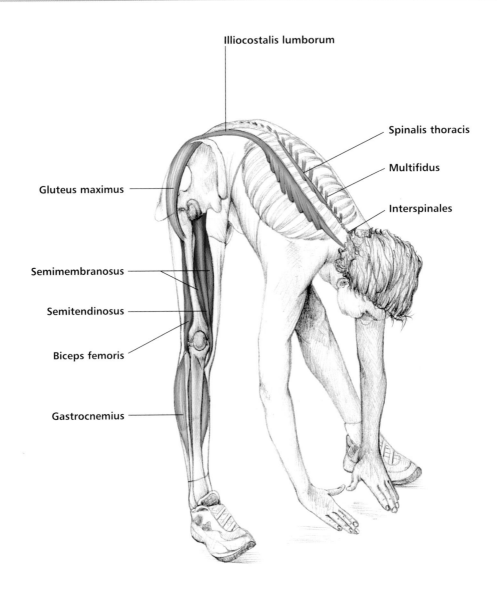

Illiocostalis lumborum

Spinalis thoracis

Multifidus

Interspinales

Gluteus maximus

Semimembranosus

Semitendinosus

Biceps femoris

Gastrocnemius

Technique
Stand with your feet shoulder-width apart. Bend forward and reach towards the ground.

Muscles being stretched
Primary muscles: Semimembranosus. Semi-tendinosus. Biceps femoris.
Secondary muscles: Gastrocnemius. Gluteus maximus. Iliocostalis lumborum. Spinalis thoracis. Interspinales. Multifidus.

Sports that benefit from this stretch
Basketball. Netball. Cycling. Hiking. Backpacking. Mountaineering. Orienteering. Ice hockey. Field hockey. Ice-skating. Roller-skating. Inline skating. Martial arts. Running. Track. Cross-country. American football (gridiron). Soccer. Rugby. Snow skiing. Water skiing. Surfing. Walking. Race walking. Wrestling.

Sports injury where stretch may be useful
Lower back muscle strain. Lower back ligament sprain. Hamstring strain. Calf strain.

Common problems and additional information for performing this stretch correctly
This position puts a lot of stress on the lower back muscles and the knees. Avoid this stretch if you have lower back pain or knee pain.

Complementary stretch
069.

13 Stretches for the Adductors

082: SITTING FEET TOGETHER ADDUCTOR STRETCH

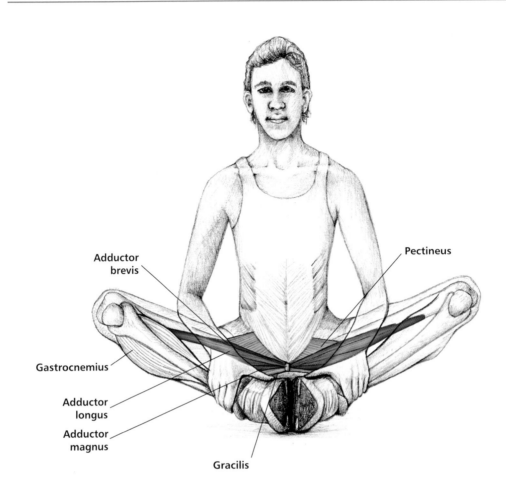

Adductor brevis

Pectineus

Gastrocnemius

Adductor longus

Adductor magnus

Gracilis

Technique
Sit with the soles of your feet together and bring your feet towards your groin. Hold onto your ankles and push your knee towards the ground with your elbows. Keep your back straight and upright.

Muscles being stretched
Primary muscles: Adductor longus, brevis and magnus.
Secondary muscles: Gracilis. Pectineus.

Sports that benefit from this stretch
Basketball. Netball. Cycling. Hiking. Backpacking. Mountaineering. Orienteering. Ice hockey. Field hockey. Ice-skating. Roller-skating. Inline skating. Martial arts. Running. Track. Cross-country. American football (gridiron). Soccer. Rugby. Snow skiing. Water skiing. Surfing. Walking. Race walking. Wrestling.

Sports injury where stretch may be useful
Avulsion fracture in the pelvic area. Groin strain. Osteitis pubis. Piriformis syndrome. Tendonitis of the adductor muscles. Trochanteric bursitis.

Additional information for performing this stretch correctly
Keep your back straight and use your elbows to regulate the intensity of this stretch.

Complementary stretch
058.

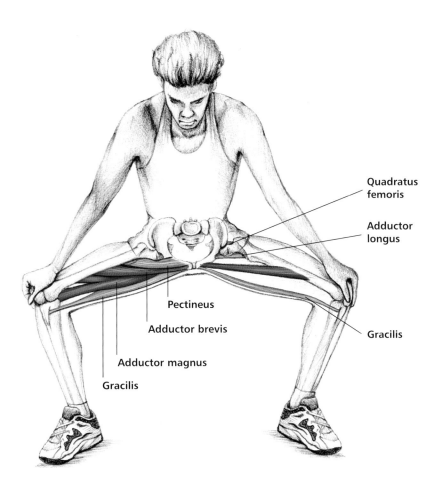

Quadratus
femoris

Adductor
longus

Pectineus

Adductor brevis

Gracilis

Adductor magnus

Gracilis

Technique
Stand with your feet wide apart and your toes pointing diagonally outwards. Bend at the knees, lean forward and use your hands to push your knees outwards.

Muscles being stretched
Primary muscles: Adductor longus, brevis and magnus.
Secondary muscles: Gracilis. Pectineus. Quadratus femoris.

Sports that benefit from this stretch
Basketball. Netball. Cycling. Hiking. Backpacking. Mountaineering. Orienteering. Ice hockey. Field hockey. Ice-skating. Roller-skating. Inline skating. Martial arts. Running. Track. Cross-country. American football (gridiron). Soccer. Rugby. Snow skiing. Water skiing. Surfing. Walking. Race walking. Wrestling.

Sports injury where stretch may be useful
Avulsion fracture in the pelvic area. Groin strain. Osteitis pubis. Piriformis syndrome. Tendonitis of the adductor muscles. Trochanteric bursitis.

Common problems and additional information for performing this stretch correctly
Holding this position for extended periods of time requires a lot of quadriceps strength. If you start to feel your legs getting weak, take a break.

Complementary stretch
087.

084: STANDING LEG-UP ADDUCTOR STRETCH

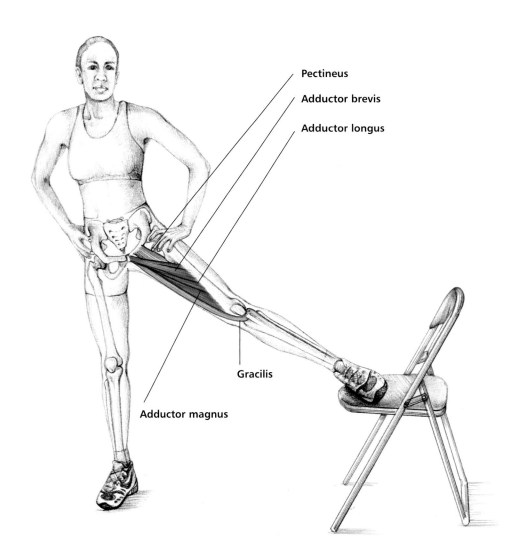

Pectineus

Adductor brevis

Adductor longus

Gracilis

Adductor magnus

Technique
Stand upright and place one leg out to the side and your foot up on a raised object. Keep your toes facing forward and slowly move your other leg away from the object.

Muscles being stretched
Primary muscles: Adductor longus, brevis and magnus.
Secondary muscles: Gracilis. Pectineus.

Sports that benefit from this stretch
Basketball. Netball. Cycling. Hiking. Backpacking. Mountaineering. Orienteering. Ice hockey. Field hockey. Ice-skating. Roller-skating. Inline skating. Martial arts. Running. Track. Cross-country. American football (gridiron). Soccer. Rugby. Snow skiing. Water skiing. Surfing. Walking. Race walking. Wrestling.

Sports injury where stretch may be useful
Avulsion fracture in the pelvic area. Groin strain. Osteitis pubis. Piriformis syndrome. Tendonitis of the adductor muscles. Trochanteric bursitis.

Additional information for performing this stretch correctly
To increase the intensity of this stretch, use a higher object and if you need to, hold onto something for balance.

Complementary stretch
082.

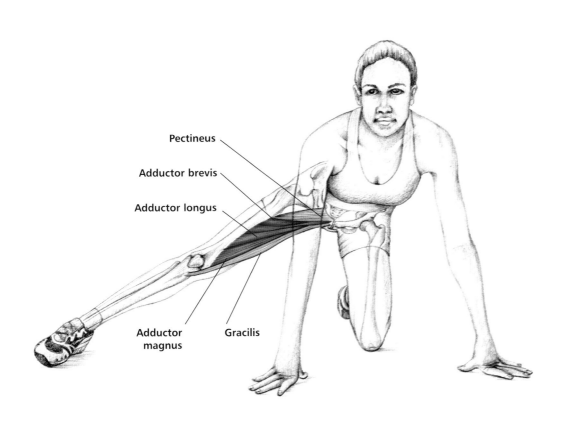

Pectineus

Adductor brevis

Adductor longus

Adductor magnus

Gracilis

Technique
Kneel on one knee and place your other leg out to the side with your toes facing forward. Rest your hands on the ground and slowly move your foot further out to the side.

Muscles being stretched
Primary muscles: Adductor longus, brevis and magnus.
Secondary muscles: Gracilis. Pectineus.

Sports that benefit from this stretch
Basketball. Netball. Cycling. Hiking. Backpacking. Mountaineering. Orienteering. Ice hockey. Field hockey. Ice-skating. Roller-skating. Inline skating. Martial arts. Running. Track. Cross-country. American football (gridiron). Soccer. Rugby. Snow skiing. Water skiing. Surfing. Walking. Race walking. Wrestling.

Sports injury where stretch may be useful
Avulsion fracture in the pelvic area. Groin strain. Osteitis pubis. Piriformis syndrome. Tendonitis of the adductor muscles. Trochanteric bursitis.

Additional information for performing this stretch correctly
If need be, place a towel or mat under your knee for comfort.

Complementary stretch
086.

086: SQUATTING LEG-OUT ADDUCTOR STRETCH

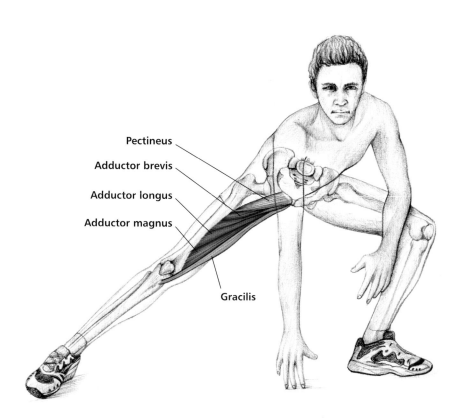

Pectineus

Adductor brevis

Adductor longus

Adductor magnus

Gracilis

Technique
Stand with your feet wide apart. Keep one leg straight and toes facing forward while bending the other leg and turning your toes out to the side. Lower your groin towards the ground and rest your hands on the bent knee or the ground.

Muscles being stretched
Primary muscles: Adductor longus, brevis and magnus.
Secondary muscles: Gracilis. Pectineus.

Sports that benefit from this stretch
Basketball. Netball. Cycling. Hiking. Backpacking. Mountaineering. Orienteering. Ice hockey. Field hockey. Ice skating. Roller skating. Inline skating. Martial arts. Running. Track. Cross country. American football (gridiron). Soccer. Rugby. Snow skiing. Water skiing. Surfing. Walking. Race walking. Wrestling.

Sports injury where stretch may be useful
Avulsion fracture in the pelvic area. Groin strain. Osteitis pubis. Piriformis syndrome. Tendonitis of the adductor muscles. Trochanteric bursitis.

Additional information for performing this stretch correctly
Increase the intensity of this stretch by lowering yourself towards the ground.

Complementary stretch
085.

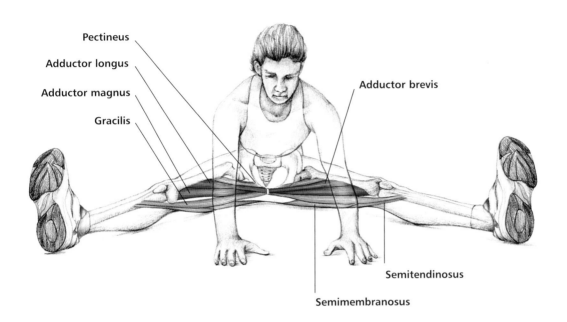

Pectineus
Adductor longus
Adductor magnus
Gracilis
Adductor brevis
Semitendinosus
Semimembranosus

Technique
Sit with your legs straight and wide apart. Keep your back straight and lean forward.

Muscles being stretched
Primary muscles: Adductor longus, brevis and magnus.
Secondary muscles: Gracilis. Pectineus. Semimembranosus. Semitendinosus.

Sports that benefit from this stretch
Basketball. Netball. Cycling. Hiking. Backpacking. Mountaineering. Orienteering. Ice hockey. Field hockey. Ice-skating. Roller-skating. Inline skating. Martial arts. Running. Track. Cross-country. American football (gridiron). Soccer. Rugby. Snow skiing. Water skiing. Surfing. Walking. Race walking. Wrestling.

Sports injury where stretch may be useful
Avulsion fracture in the pelvic area. Groin strain. Osteitis pubis. Piriformis syndrome. Tendonitis of the adductor muscles. Trochanteric bursitis. Hamstring strain.

Additional information for performing this stretch correctly
To increase the intensity of this stretch, move your legs further apart.

Complementary stretch
086.

088: STANDING WIDE LEG ADDUCTOR STRETCH

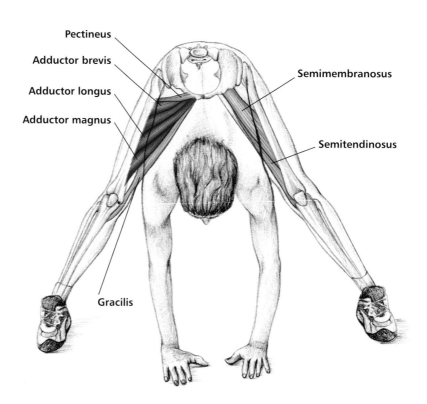

Pectineus
Adductor brevis
Adductor longus
Adductor magnus
Semimembranosus
Semitendinosus
Gracilis

Technique
Stand with your feet wide apart and your toes facing forward. Lean forward and reach towards the ground.

Muscles being stretched
Primary muscles: Adductor longus, brevis and magnus.
Secondary muscles: Gracilis. Pectineus. Semimembranosus. Semitendinosus.

Sports that benefit from this stretch
Basketball. Netball. Cycling. Hiking. Backpacking. Mountaineering. Orienteering. Ice hockey. Field hockey. Ice-skating. Roller-skating. Inline skating. Martial arts. Running. Track. Cross-country. American football (gridiron). Soccer. Rugby. Snow skiing. Water skiing. Surfing. Walking. Race walking. Wrestling.

Sports injury where stretch may be useful
Avulsion fracture in the pelvic area. Groin strain. Osteitis pubis. Piriformis syndrome. Tendonitis of the adductor muscles. Trochanteric bursitis. Hamstring strain.

Common problems and additional information for performing this stretch correctly
This position puts a lot of stress on the lower back muscles and the knees. Avoid this stretch if you have lower back pain or knee pain.

Complementary stretch
084.

14

Stretches for the Abductors

089: STANDING HIP-OUT ABDUCTOR STRETCH

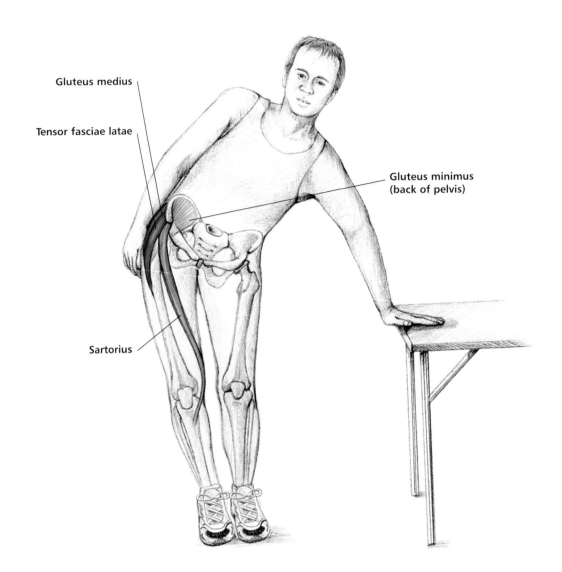

Gluteus medius

Tensor fasciae latae

Gluteus minimus
(back of pelvis)

Sartorius

Technique
Stand upright beside a wall or table with both feet together. Lean your upper body towards the wall and push your hips away from the wall. Keep your outside leg straight and your inside leg slightly bent.

Muscles being stretched
Primary muscles: Tensor fasciae latae. Gluteus medius and minimus.
Secondary muscle: Sartorius.

Sports that benefit from this stretch
Basketball. Netball. Cycling. Hiking. Backpacking. Mountaineering. Orienteering. Ice hockey. Field hockey. Ice-skating. Roller-skating. Inline skating. Martial arts. Running. Track. Cross-country. American football (gridiron). Soccer. Rugby. Snow skiing. Water skiing. Surfing. Walking. Race walking. Wrestling.

Sports injury where stretch may be useful
Trochanteric bursitis. Iliotibial band syndrome.

Common problems and additional information for performing this stretch correctly
It is important not to bend forward during this stretch. Keep your body upright and concentrate on pushing your hips away from the object you're leaning on.

Complementary stretch
092.

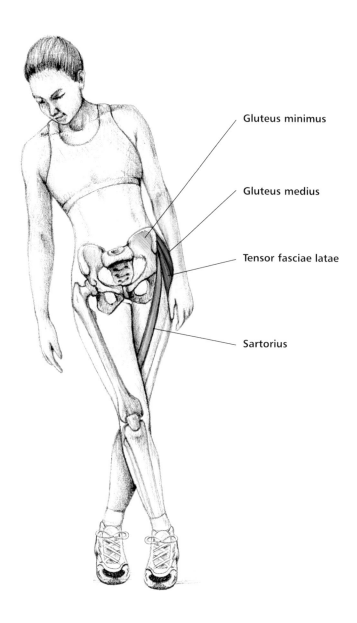

Gluteus minimus

Gluteus medius

Tensor fasciae latae

Sartorius

Technique
Stand upright and cross one foot behind the other. Lean towards the foot that is behind the other.

Muscles being stretched
Primary muscles: Tensor fasciae latae. Gluteus medius and minimus.
Secondary muscle: Sartorius.

Sports that benefit from this stretch
Basketball. Netball. Cycling. Hiking. Backpacking. Mountaineering. Orienteering. Ice hockey. Field hockey. Ice-skating. Roller-skating. Inline skating. Martial arts. Running. Track. Cross-country. American football (gridiron). Soccer. Rugby. Snow skiing. Water skiing. Surfing. Walking. Race walking. Wrestling.

Sports injury where stretch may be useful
Trochanteric bursitis. Iliotibial band syndrome.

Additional information for performing this stretch correctly
If need be, hold onto something for balance. This will allow you to concentrate on the stretch, instead of worrying about falling over.

Complementary stretch
049.

091: STANDING LEG-UNDER ABDUCTOR STRETCH

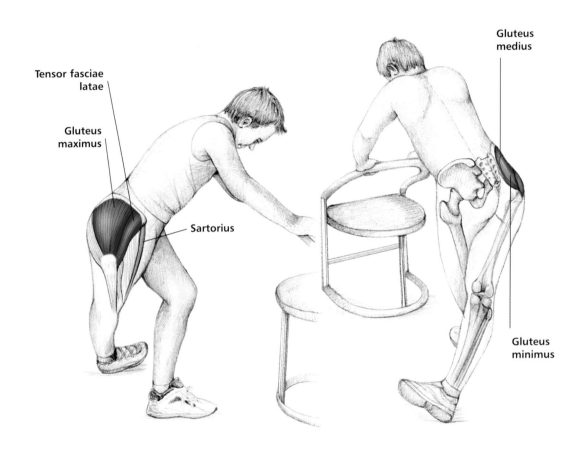

Tensor fasciae latae

Gluteus maximus

Sartorius

Gluteus medius

Gluteus minimus

Technique
While standing, lean forward and hold onto a chair or bench to help with balance. Cross one foot behind the other and slide that foot away from your body, keeping your leg straight. Slowly bend your front leg to lower your body.

Muscles being stretched
Primary muscles: Tensor fasciae latae. Gluteus medius and mininus.
Secondary muscle: Sartorius.

Sports that benefit from this stretch
Basketball. Netball. Cycling. Hiking. Backpacking. Mountaineering. Orienteering. Ice hockey. Field hockey. Ice-skating. Roller-skating. Inline skating. Martial arts. Running. Track. Cross-country. American football (gridiron). Soccer. Rugby. Snow skiing. Water skiing. Surfing. Walking. Race walking. Wrestling.

Sports injury where stretch may be useful
Trochanteric bursitis. Iliotibial band syndrome.

Additional information for performing this stretch correctly
Regulate the intensity of the stretch by using your bent leg to lower your body.

Complementary stretch
090.

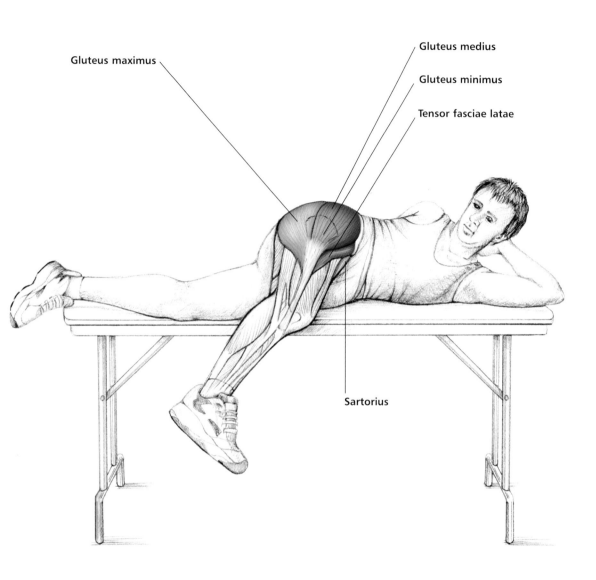

Gluteus maximus

Gluteus medius

Gluteus minimus

Tensor fasciae latae

Sartorius

Technique
Lie on a bench on your side. Allow the top leg to fall forward and off the side of the bench.

Muscles being stretched
Primary muscles: Tensor fasciae latae. Gluteus medius and mininus.
Secondary muscles: Sartorius. Gluteus maximus.

Sports that benefit from this stretch
Basketball. Netball. Cycling. Hiking. Backpacking. Mountaineering. Orienteering. Ice hockey. Field hockey. Ice-skating. Roller-skating. Inline skating. Martial arts. Running. Track. Cross-country. American football (gridiron). Soccer. Rugby. Snow skiing. Water skiing. Surfing. Walking. Race walking. Wrestling.

Sports injury where stretch may be useful
Trochanteric bursitis. Iliotibial band syndrome.

Common problems and additional information for performing this stretch correctly
Try not to let your leg fall too far forward and use the weight of your leg to do the stretching for you.

Complementary stretch
059.

15 Stretches for the Calves

093: STANDING TOE-UP CALF STRETCH

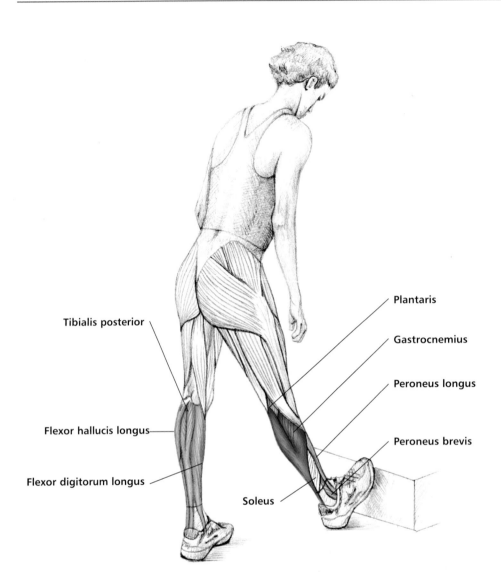

Tibialis posterior

Flexor hallucis longus

Flexor digitorum longus

Plantaris

Gastrocnemius

Peroneus longus

Peroneus brevis

Soleus

Technique
Stand upright and place your toes on a step or raised object. Keep your leg straight and lean towards your toes.

Muscles being stretched
Primary muscle: Gastrocnemius.
Secondary muscles: Tibialis posterior. Flexor hallucis longus. Flexor digitorum longus. Peroneus longus and brevis. Plantaris.

Sports that benefit from this stretch
Basketball. Netball. Boxing. Cycling. Hiking. Backpacking. Mountaineering. Orienteering. Ice hockey. Field hockey. Ice-skating. Roller-skating. Inline skating. Martial arts. Tennis. Badminton. Squash. Running. Track. Cross-country. American football (gridiron). Soccer. Rugby. Snow skiing. Water skiing. Surfing. Swimming. Walking. Race walking.

Sports injury where stretch may be useful
Calf strain. Achilles tendon strain. Achilles tendonitis. Medial tibial pain syndrome (shin splints).

Additional information for performing this stretch correctly
Regulate the intensity of this stretch by keeping your back straight and leaning forward.

Complementary stretch
095.

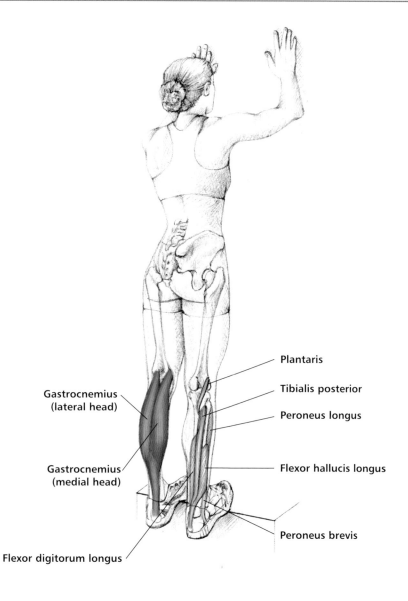

Plantaris

Tibialis posterior

Peroneus longus

Gastrocnemius
(lateral head)

Flexor hallucis longus

Gastrocnemius
(medial head)

Peroneus brevis

Flexor digitorum longus

Technique
Stand on a raised object or step. Put the toes of both of your feet on the edge of the step and keep your legs straight. Let your heels drop towards the ground and lean forward.

Muscles being stretched
Primary muscle: Gastrocnemius.
Secondary muscles: Tibialis posterior. Flexor hallucis longus. Flexor digitorum longus. Peroneus longus and brevis. Plantaris.

Sports that benefit from this stretch
Basketball. Netball. Boxing. Cycling. Hiking. Backpacking. Mountaineering. Orienteering. Ice hockey. Field hockey. Ice-skating. Roller-skating. Inline skating. Martial arts. Tennis. Badminton. Squash. Running. Track. Cross-country. American football (gridiron). Soccer. Rugby. Snow skiing. Water skiing. Surfing. Swimming. Walking. Race walking.

Sports injury where stretch may be useful
Calf strain. Achilles tendon strain. Achilles tendonitis. Medial tibial pain syndrome (shin splints).

Additional information for performing this stretch correctly
Let your body weight regulate the intensity of this stretch.

Complementary stretch
097.

095: SINGLE HEEL DROP CALF STRETCH

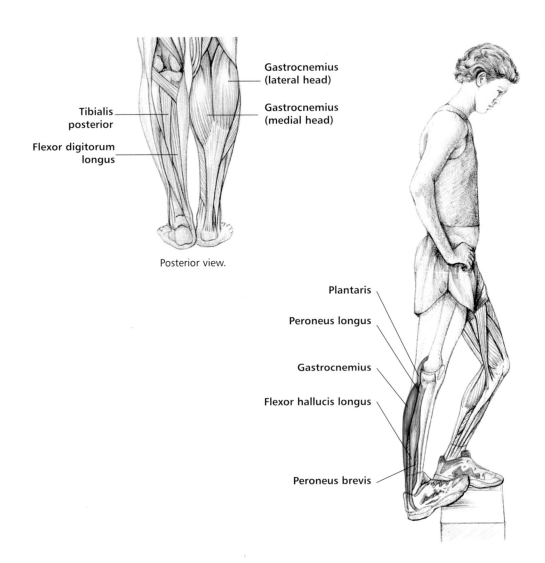

Gastrocnemius (lateral head)

Gastrocnemius (medial head)

Tibialis posterior

Flexor digitorum longus

Posterior view.

Plantaris

Peroneus longus

Gastrocnemius

Flexor hallucis longus

Peroneus brevis

Technique
Stand on a raised object or step. Put the toes of one foot on the edge of the step and keep your leg straight. Let your heel drop towards the ground.

Muscles being stretched
Primary muscle: Gastrocnemius.
Secondary muscles: Tibialis posterior. Flexor hallucis longus. Flexor digitorum longus. Peroneus longus and brevis. Plantaris.

Sports that benefit from this stretch
Basketball. Netball. Boxing. Cycling. Hiking. Backpacking. Mountaineering. Orienteering. Ice hockey. Field hockey. Ice-skating. Roller-skating. Inline skating. Martial arts. Tennis. Badminton. Squash. Running. Track. Cross-country. American football (gridiron). Soccer. Rugby. Snow skiing. Water skiing. Surfing. Swimming. Walking. Race walking.

Sports injury where stretch may be useful
Calf strain. Achilles tendon strain. Achilles tendonitis. Medial tibial pain syndrome (shin splints).

Common problems and additional information for performing this stretch correctly
This stretch can put a lot of pressure on the Achilles tendon. Ease into this stretch by slowly lowering your heel.

Complementary stretch
099.

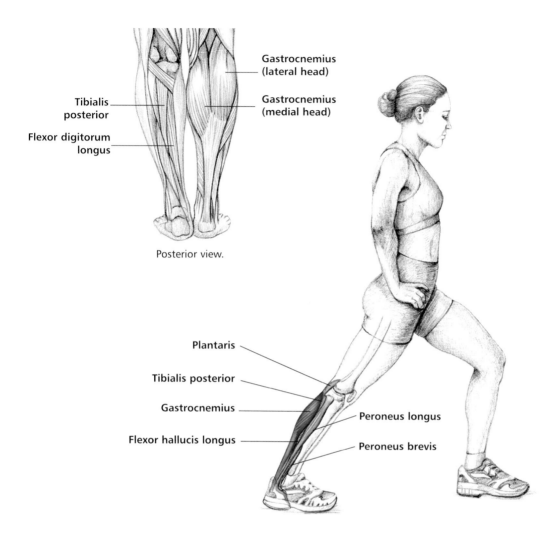

Posterior view.

Technique
Stand upright and then take one big step backwards. Keep your back leg straight and push your heel to the ground.

Muscles being stretched
Primary muscle: Gastrocnemius.
Secondary muscles: Tibialis posterior. Flexor hallucis longus. Flexor digitorum longus. Peroneus longus and brevis. Plantaris.

Sports that benefit from this stretch
Basketball. Netball. Boxing. Cycling. Hiking. Backpacking. Mountaineering. Orienteering. Ice hockey. Field hockey. Ice-skating. Roller-skating. Inline skating. Martial arts. Tennis. Badminton. Squash. Running. Track. Cross-country. American football (gridiron). Soccer. Rugby. Snow skiing. Water skiing. Surfing. Swimming. Walking. Race walking.

Sports injury where stretch may be useful
Calf strain. Achilles tendon strain. Achilles tendonitis. Medial tibial pain syndrome (shin splints).

Common problems and additional information for performing this stretch correctly
Make sure that the toes of your back leg are facing forward. Letting your toes point to one side will cause this stretch to put uneven tension on the calf muscles. Over an extended period of time, this could lead to a muscle imbalance.

Complementary stretch
093.

STRETCHES FOR THE CALVES

097: LEANING HEEL BACK CALF STRETCH

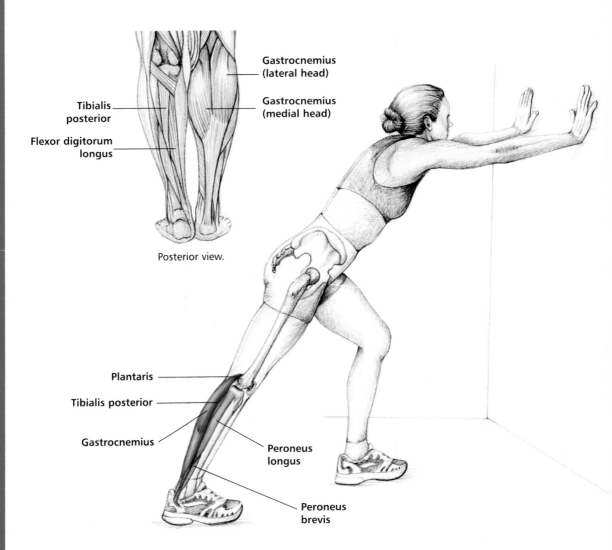

Gastrocnemius (lateral head)

Gastrocnemius (medial head)

Tibialis posterior

Flexor digitorum longus

Posterior view.

Plantaris

Tibialis posterior

Gastrocnemius

Peroneus longus

Peroneus brevis

Technique
Stand upright and lean against a wall. Place one foot as far from the wall as is comfortable and make sure that both toes are facing forward and your heel is on the ground. Keep your back leg straight and lean towards the wall.

Muscles being stretched
Primary muscle: Gastrocnemius.
Secondary muscles: Tibialis posterior. Flexor hallucis longus. Flexor digitorum longus. Peroneus longus and brevis. Plantaris.

Sports that benefit from this stretch
Basketball. Netball. Boxing. Cycling. Hiking. Backpacking. Mountaineering. Orienteering. Ice hockey. Field hockey. Ice-skating. Roller-skating. Inline skating. Martial arts. Tennis. Badminton. Squash. Running. Track. Cross-country. American football (gridiron). Soccer. Rugby. Snow skiing. Water skiing. Surfing. Swimming. Walking. Race walking.

Sports injury where stretch may be useful
Calf strain. Achilles tendon strain. Achilles tendonitis. Medial tibial pain syndrome (shin splints).

Common problems and additional information for performing this stretch correctly
Make sure the toes of your back leg are facing forward. Letting your toes point to one side will cause this stretch to put uneven tension on the calf muscles. Over an extended period of time, this could lead to a muscle imbalance.

Complementary stretch
099.

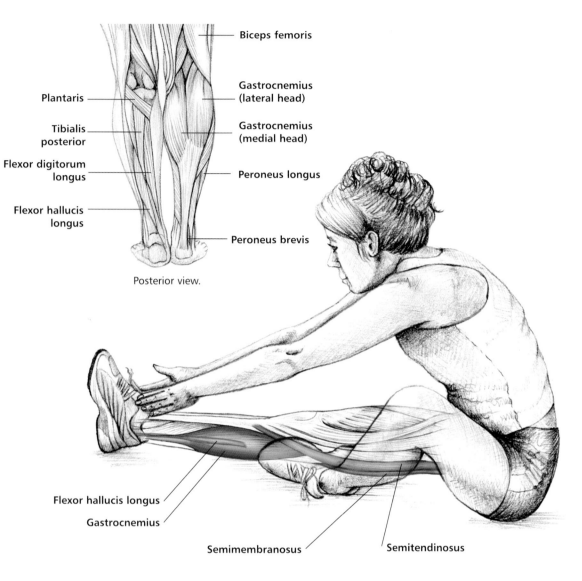

Biceps femoris

Gastrocnemius
(lateral head)

Plantaris

Gastrocnemius
(medial head)

Tibialis
posterior

Flexor digitorum
longus

Peroneus longus

Flexor hallucis
longus

Peroneus brevis

Posterior view.

Flexor hallucis longus

Gastrocnemius

Semimembranosus

Semitendinosus

Technique
Sit with one leg straight and your toes pointing up. Lean forward and pull your toes back towards your body.

Muscles being stretched
Primary muscles: Gastrocnemius. Semi-membranosus. Semitendinosus. Biceps femoris. Secondary muscles: Tibialis posterior. Flexor hallucis longus. Flexor digitorum longus. Peroneus longus and brevis. Plantaris.

Sports that benefit from this stretch
Basketball. Netball. Boxing. Cycling. Hiking. Backpacking. Mountaineering. Orienteering. Ice hockey. Field hockey. Ice-skating. Roller-skating. Inline skating. Martial arts. Tennis. Badminton. Squash. Running. Track. Cross-country. American football (gridiron). Soccer. Rugby. Snow skiing. Water skiing. Surfing. Swimming. Walking. Race walking.

Sports injury where stretch may be useful
Hamstring strain. Calf strain. Achilles tendon strain. Achilles tendonitis. Medial tibial pain syndrome (shin splints).

Common problems and additional information for performing this stretch correctly
If you have trouble reaching your toes in this position, avoid this stretch.

Complementary stretch
100.

099: STANDING TOE RAISED CALF STRETCH

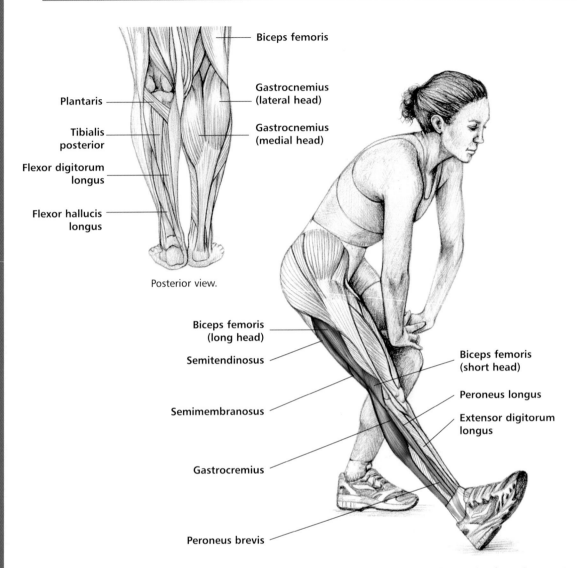

Biceps femoris
Gastrocnemius (lateral head)
Plantaris
Gastrocnemius (medial head)
Tibialis posterior
Flexor digitorum longus
Flexor hallucis longus

Posterior view.

Biceps femoris (long head)
Semitendinosus
Biceps femoris (short head)
Peroneus longus
Semimembranosus
Extensor digitorum longus
Gastrocremius
Peroneus brevis

Technique
Stand with one knee bent and the other leg straight out in front. Point your toes towards your body and lean forward. Keep your back straight and rest your hands on your bent knee.

Muscles being stretched
Primary muscles: Gastrocnemius. Semi-membranosus. Semitendinosus. Biceps femoris. Secondary muscles: Tibialis posterior. Flexor hallucis longus. Flexor digitorum longus. Peroneus longus and brevis. Plantaris.

Sports that benefit from this stretch
Basketball. Netball. Boxing. Cycling. Hiking. Backpacking. Mountaineering. Orienteering. Ice hockey. Field hockey. Ice-skating. Roller-skating. Inline skating. Martial arts. Tennis. Badminton. Squash. Running. Track. Cross-country. American football (gridiron). Soccer. Rugby. Snow skiing. Water skiing. Surfing. Swimming. Walking. Race walking.

Sports injury where stretch may be useful
Hamstring strain. Calf strain. Achilles tendon strain. Achilles tendonitis. Medial tibial pain syndrome (shin splints).

Common problems and additional information for performing this stretch correctly
Make sure your toes are pointing upward. Letting your toes point to one side will cause this stretch to put uneven tension on the calf muscles. Over an extended period of time, this could lead to a muscle imbalance.

Complementary stretch
094.

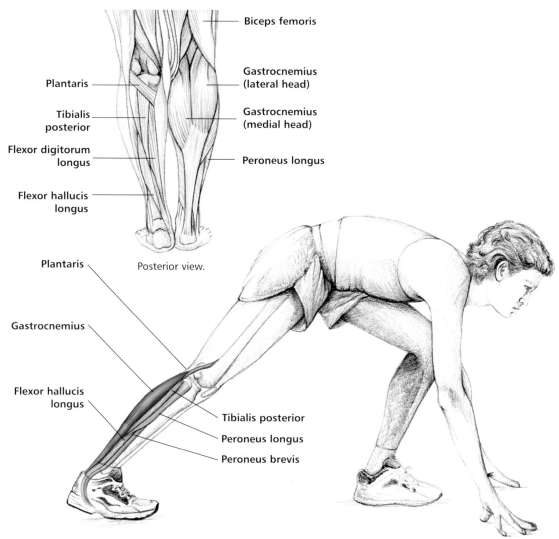

Biceps femoris

Gastrocnemius (lateral head)

Plantaris

Gastrocnemius (medial head)

Tibialis posterior

Flexor digitorum longus

Peroneus longus

Flexor hallucis longus

Plantaris

Posterior view.

Gastrocnemius

Flexor hallucis longus

Tibialis posterior

Peroneus longus

Peroneus brevis

Technique
Stand upright and place one foot in front of the other. Bend your front leg and keep your back leg straight. Push your heel to the ground and lean forward. Place your hands on the ground in front of you.

Muscles being stretched
Primary muscle: Gastrocnemius.
Secondary muscles: Tibialis posterior. Flexor hallucis longus. Flexor digitorum longus. Peroneus longus and brevis. Plantaris.

Sports that benefit from this stretch
Basketball. Netball. Boxing. Cycling. Hiking. Backpacking. Mountaineering. Orienteering. Ice hockey. Field hockey. Ice-skating. Roller-skating. Inline skating. Martial arts. Tennis. Badminton. Squash. Running. Track. Cross-country. American football (gridiron). Soccer. Rugby. Snow skiing. Water skiing. Surfing. Swimming. Walking. Race walking.

Sports injury where stretch may be useful
Calf strain. Achilles tendon strain. Achilles tendonitis. Medial tibial pain syndrome (shin splints).

Common problems and additional information for performing this stretch correctly
Make sure the toes of your back leg are facing forward. Letting your toes point to one side will cause this stretch to put uneven tension on the calf muscles. Over an extended period of time, this could lead to a muscle imbalance.

Complementary stretch
098.

101: STANDING TOE-UP ACHILLES STRETCH

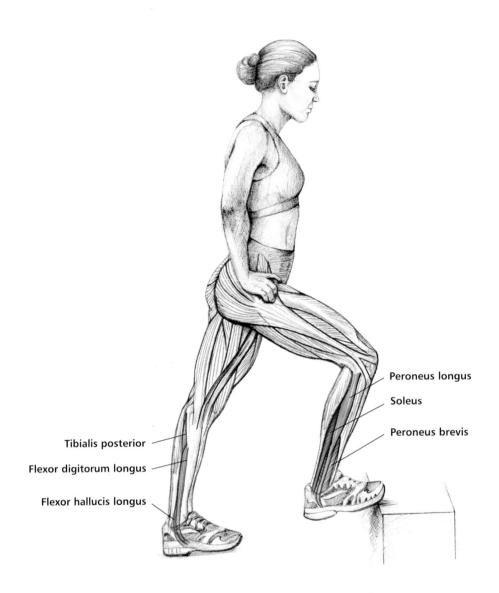

Peroneus longus

Soleus

Peroneus brevis

Tibialis posterior

Flexor digitorum longus

Flexor hallucis longus

Technique
Stand upright and place your toes against a step or raised object. Bend your leg and lean towards your toes.

Muscles being stretched
Primary muscle: Soleus.
Secondary muscles: Tibialis posterior. Flexor hallucis longus. Flexor digitorum longus. Peroneus longus and brevis.

Sports that benefit from this stretch
Basketball. Netball. Boxing. Cycling. Hiking. Backpacking. Mountaineering. Orienteering. Ice hockey. Field hockey. Ice-skating. Roller-skating. Inline skating. Martial arts. Tennis. Badminton. Squash. Running. Track. Cross-country. American football (gridiron). Soccer. Rugby. Snow skiing. Water skiing. Surfing. Swimming. Walking. Race walking.

Sports injury where stretch may be useful
Calf strain. Achilles tendon strain. Achilles tendonitis. Medial tibial pain syndrome (shin splints). Posterior tibial tendonitis.

Additional information for performing this stretch correctly
Regulate the intensity of this stretch by relaxing your calf muscles and pushing your heel to the ground.

Complementary stretch
103.

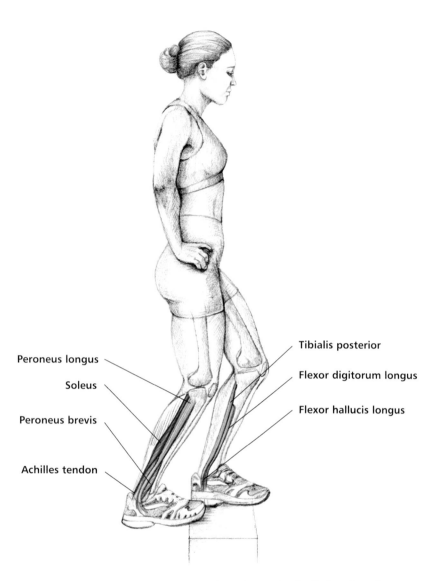

Peroneus longus

Soleus

Peroneus brevis

Achilles tendon

Tibialis posterior

Flexor digitorum longus

Flexor hallucis longus

Technique
Stand on a raised object or step and place the toes of one of your feet on the edge of the step. Bend your leg and let your heel drop towards the ground.

Muscles being stretched
Primary muscle: Soleus.
Secondary muscles: Tibialis posterior. Flexor hallucis longus. Flexor digitorum longus. Peroneus longus and brevis.

Sports that benefit from this stretch
Basketball. Netball. Boxing. Cycling. Hiking. Backpacking. Mountaineering. Orienteering. Ice hockey. Field hockey. Ice-skating. Roller-skating. Inline skating. Martial arts. Tennis. Badminton. Squash. Running. Track. Cross-country. American football (gridiron). Soccer. Rugby. Snow skiing. Water skiing. Surfing. Swimming. Walking. Race walking.

Sports injury where stretch may be useful
Calf strain. Achilles tendon strain. Achilles tendonitis. Medial tibial pain syndrome (shin splints). Posterior tibial tendonitis.

Common problems and additional information for performing this stretch correctly
This stretch can put a lot of pressure on the Achilles tendon. Ease into this stretch by slowly lowering your heel.

Complementary stretch
104.

103: STANDING HEEL BACK ACHILLES STRETCH

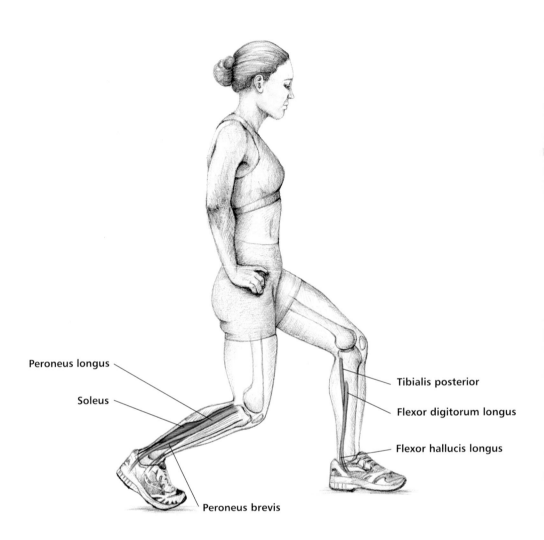

Peroneus longus

Soleus

Tibialis posterior

Flexor digitorum longus

Flexor hallucis longus

Peroneus brevis

Technique
Stand upright and take one big step backwards. Bend your back leg and push your heel towards the ground.

Muscles being stretched
Primary muscle: Soleus.
Secondary muscles: Tibialis posterior. Flexor hallucis longus. Flexor digitorum longus. Peroneus longus and brevis.

Sports that benefit from this stretch
Basketball. Netball. Boxing. Cycling. Hiking. Backpacking. Mountaineering. Orienteering. Ice hockey. Field hockey. Ice-skating. Roller-skating. Inline skating. Martial arts. Tennis. Badminton. Squash. Running. Track. Cross-country. American football (gridiron). Soccer. Rugby. Snow skiing. Water skiing. Surfing. Swimming. Walking. Race walking.

Sports injury where stretch may be useful
Calf strain. Achilles tendon strain. Achilles tendonitis. Medial tibial pain syndrome (shin splints). Posterior tibial tendonitis.

Common problems and additional information for performing this stretch correctly
Make sure the toes of your back leg are facing forward. Letting your toes point to one side will cause this stretch to put uneven tension on the calf muscles. Over an extended period of time, this could lead to a muscle imbalance. Regulate the intensity of this stretch by lowering your body.

Complementary stretch
105.

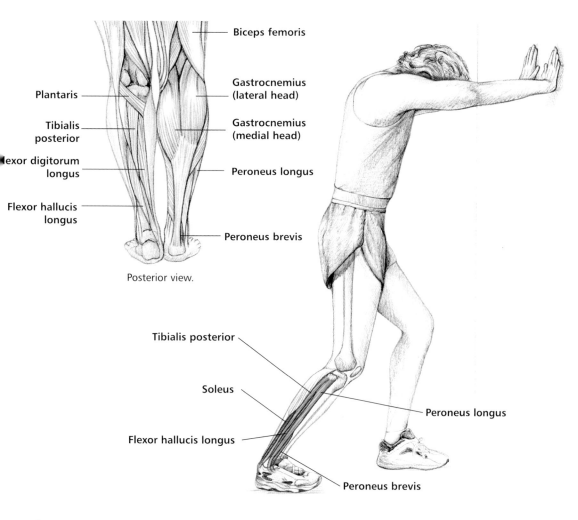

Biceps femoris

Gastrocnemius (lateral head)

Plantaris

Gastrocnemius (medial head)

Tibialis posterior

Flexor digitorum longus

Peroneus longus

Flexor hallucis longus

Peroneus brevis

Posterior view.

Tibialis posterior

Soleus

Flexor hallucis longus

Peroneus longus

Peroneus brevis

Technique
Stand upright while leaning against a wall and place one foot behind the other. Make sure that both toes are facing forward and your heel is on the ground. Bend your back leg and lean towards the wall.

Muscles being stretched
Primary muscle: Soleus.
Secondary muscles: Tibialis posterior. Flexor hallucis longus. Flexor digitorum longus. Peroneus longus and brevis.

Sports that benefit from this stretch
Basketball. Netball. Boxing. Cycling. Hiking. Backpacking. Mountaineering. Orienteering. Ice hockey. Field hockey. Ice-skating. Roller-skating. Inline skating. Martial arts. Tennis. Badminton. Squash. Running. Track. Cross-country. American football (gridiron). Soccer. Rugby. Snow skiing. Water skiing. Surfing. Swimming. Walking. Race walking.

Sports injury where stretch may be useful
Calf strain. Achilles tendon strain. Achilles tendonitis. Medial tibial pain syndrome (shin splints). Posterior tibial tendonitis.

Common problems and additional information for performing this stretch correctly
Make sure the toes of your back leg are facing forward. Letting your toes point to one side will cause this stretch to put uneven tension on the calf muscles. Over an extended period of time, this could lead to a muscle imbalance. Regulate the intensity of this stretch by lowering your body.

Complementary stretch
102.

105: SITTING BENT KNEE TOE PULL ACHILLES STRETCH

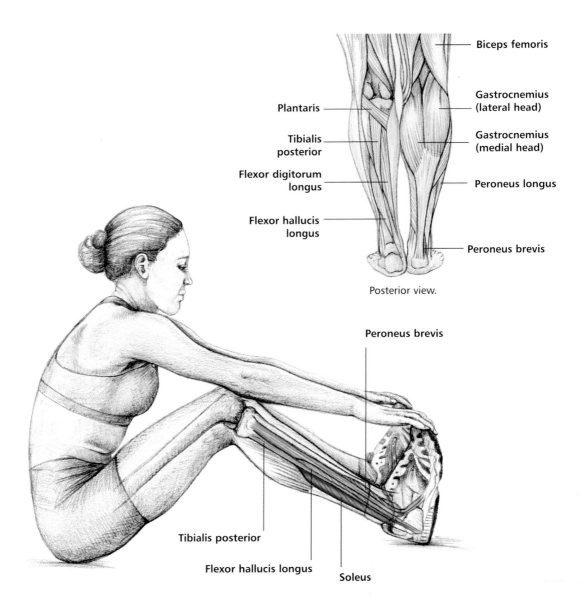

Biceps femoris

Plantaris

Gastrocnemius (lateral head)

Tibialis posterior

Gastrocnemius (medial head)

Flexor digitorum longus

Peroneus longus

Flexor hallucis longus

Peroneus brevis

Posterior view.

Peroneus brevis

Tibialis posterior

Flexor hallucis longus

Soleus

Technique
Sit with your legs out in front and bend both knees. Grab hold of your toes and pull them towards your knees.

Muscles being stretched
Primary muscle: Soleus.
Secondary muscles: Tibialis posterior. Flexor hallucis longus. Flexor digitorum longus. Peroneus longus and brevis.

Sports that benefit from this stretch
Basketball. Netball. Boxing. Cycling. Hiking. Backpacking. Mountaineering. Orienteering. Ice hockey. Field hockey. Ice-skating. Roller-skating. Inline skating. Martial arts. Tennis. Badminton. Squash. Running. Track. Cross-country. American football (gridiron). Soccer. Rugby. Snow skiing. Water skiing. Surfing. Swimming. Walking. Race walking.

Sports injury where stretch may be useful
Calf strain. Achilles tendon strain. Achilles tendonitis. Medial tibial pain syndrome (shin splints). Posterior tibial tendonitis.

Additional information for performing this stretch correctly
Regulate the intensity of this stretch by pushing your heels forward and pulling your toes back.

Complementary stretch
101.

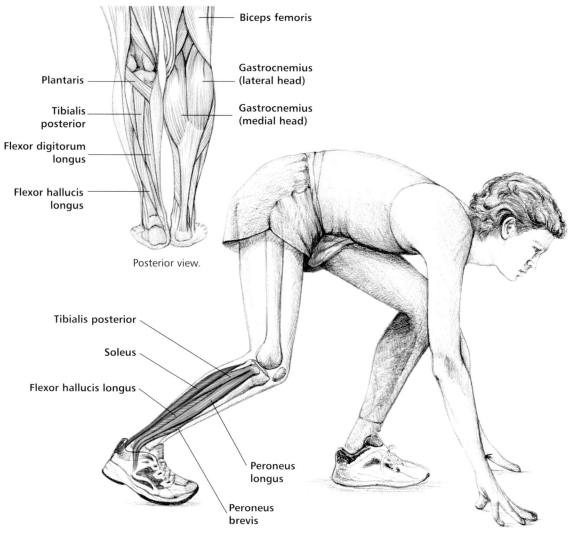

Biceps femoris

Gastrocnemius
(lateral head)

Plantaris

Gastrocnemius
(medial head)

Tibialis
posterior

Flexor digitorum
longus

Flexor hallucis
longus

Posterior view.

Tibialis posterior

Soleus

Flexor hallucis longus

Peroneus
longus

Peroneus
brevis

Technique
Stand upright and place one foot in front of the other. Bend both your front leg and your back leg and then push your back heel towards the ground. Lean forward and place your hands on the ground in front of you.

Muscles being stretched
Primary muscle: Soleus.
Secondary muscles: Tibialis posterior. Flexor hallucis longus. Flexor digitorum longus. Peroneus longus and brevis.

Sports that benefit from this stretch
Basketball. Netball. Boxing. Cycling. Hiking. Backpacking. Mountaineering. Orienteering. Ice hockey. Field hockey. Ice-skating. Roller-skating. Inline skating. Martial arts. Tennis. Badminton. Squash. Running. Track. Cross-country. American football (gridiron). Soccer. Rugby.

Snow skiing. Water skiing. Surfing. Swimming. Walking. Race walking.

Sports injury where stretch may be useful
Calf strain. Achilles tendon strain. Achilles tendonitis. Medial tibial pain syndrome (shin splints). Posterior tibial tendonitis.

Common problems and additional information for performing this stretch correctly
Make sure the toes of your back leg are facing forward. Letting your toes point to one side will cause this stretch to put uneven tension on the calf muscles. Over an extended period of time, this could lead to a muscle imbalance.

Complementary stretch
104.

107: KNEELING HEEL-DOWN ACHILLES STRETCH

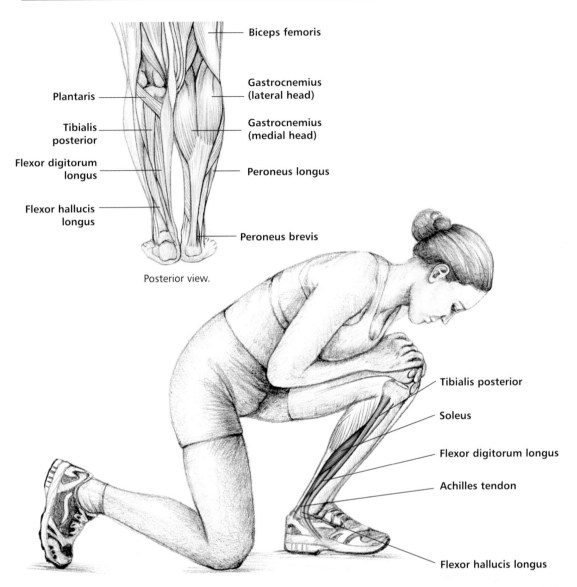

Biceps femoris

Gastrocnemius (lateral head)

Plantaris

Tibialis posterior

Gastrocnemius (medial head)

Flexor digitorum longus

Peroneus longus

Flexor hallucis longus

Peroneus brevis

Posterior view.

Tibialis posterior

Soleus

Flexor digitorum longus

Achilles tendon

Flexor hallucis longus

Technique
Kneel on one foot and place your body weight over your knee. Keep your heel on the ground and lean forward.

Muscles being stretched
Primary muscle: Soleus.
Secondary muscles: Tibialis posterior. Flexor hallucis longus. Flexor digitorum longus. Peroneus longus and brevis.

Sports that benefit from this stretch
Basketball. Netball. Boxing. Cycling. Hiking. Backpacking. Mountaineering. Orienteering. Ice hockey. Field hockey. Ice-skating. Roller-skating. Inline skating. Martial arts. Tennis. Badminton. Squash. Running. Track. Cross-country. American football (gridiron). Soccer. Rugby. Snow skiing. Water skiing. Surfing. Swimming. Walking. Race walking.

Sports injury where stretch may be useful
Calf strain. Achilles tendon strain. Achilles tendonitis. Medial tibial pain syndrome (shin splints). Posterior tibial tendonitis.

Common problems and additional information for performing this stretch correctly
This stretch can put a lot of pressure on the Achilles tendon. Ease into this stretch by slowly leaning forward.

Complementary stretch
101.

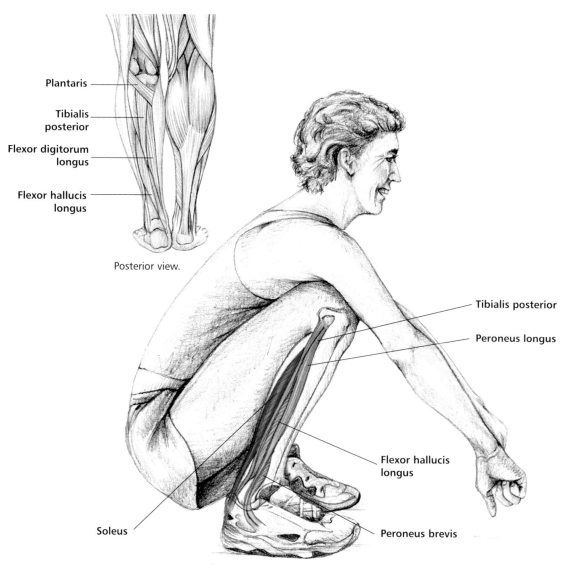

Plantaris

Tibialis posterior

Flexor digitorum longus

Flexor hallucis longus

Posterior view.

Tibialis posterior

Peroneus longus

Flexor hallucis longus

Peroneus brevis

Soleus

Technique
Stand with your feet at shoulder-width apart. Bend your legs and lower to a sitting position. Place your hands out in front for balance.

Muscles being stretched
Primary muscle: Soleus.
Secondary muscles: Tibialis posterior. Flexor hallucis longus. Flexor digitorum longus. Peroneus longus and brevis.

Sports that benefit from this stretch
Basketball. Netball. Boxing. Cycling. Hiking. Backpacking. Mountaineering. Orienteering. Ice hockey. Field hockey. Ice-skating. Roller-skating. Inline skating. Martial arts. Tennis. Badminton. Squash. Running. Track. Cross-country. American football (gridiron). Soccer. Rugby. Snow skiing. Water skiing. Surfing. Swimming. Walking. Race walking.

Sports injury where stretch may be useful
Calf strain. Achilles tendon strain. Achilles tendonitis. Medial tibial pain syndrome (shin splints). Posterior tibial tendonitis.

Additional information for performing this stretch correctly
If need be, hold onto something for balance and make sure your toes are facing forward.

Complementary stretch
107.

16

Stretches for the Shins, Ankles and Feet

109: FOOT-BEHIND SHIN STRETCH

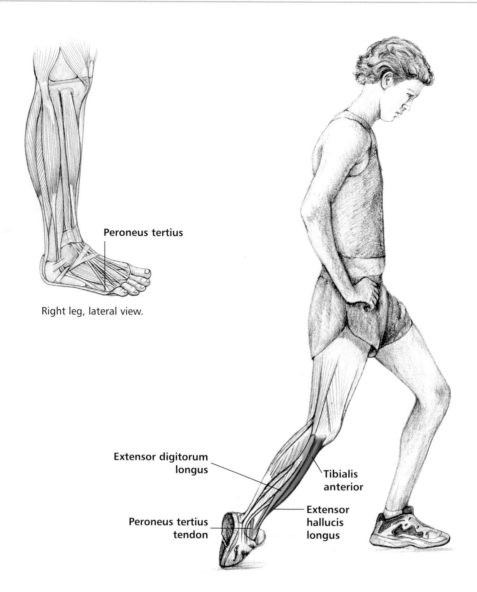

Peroneus tertius

Right leg, lateral view.

Extensor digitorum longus

Tibialis anterior

Peroneus tertius tendon

Extensor hallucis longus

Technique
Stand upright and place the top of your toes on the ground behind you. Push your ankle to the ground.

Muscles being stretched
Primary muscle: Tibialis anterior.
Secondary muscles: Extensor hallucis longus. Extensor digitorum longus. Peroneus tertius.

Sports that benefit from this stretch
Basketball. Netball. Boxing. Hiking. Backpacking. Mountaineering. Orienteering. Martial arts. Tennis. Badminton. Squash. Running. Track. Cross-country. American football (gridiron). Soccer. Rugby. Walking. Race walking.

Sports injury where stretch may be useful
Anterior compartment syndrome. Medial tibial pain syndrome (shin splints). Ankle sprain. Peroneal tendon subluxation. Peroneal tendonitis.

Additional information for performing this stretch correctly
Regulate the intensity of this stretch by lowering your body and pushing your ankle to the ground. If need be, hold onto something for balance.

Complementary stretch
111.

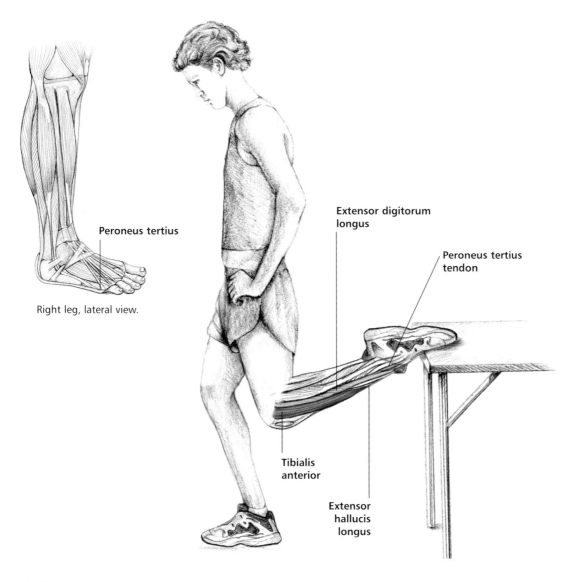

Peroneus tertius

Right leg, lateral view.

Extensor digitorum longus

Peroneus tertius tendon

Tibialis anterior

Extensor hallucis longus

Technique
Stand upright and place the top of your toes on a raised object behind you. Push your ankle downwards.

Muscles being stretched
Primary muscle: Tibialis anterior.
Secondary muscles: Extensor hallucis longus. Extensor digitorum longus. Peroneus tertius.

Sports that benefit from this stretch
Basketball. Netball. Boxing. Hiking. Backpacking. Mountaineering. Orienteering. Martial arts. Tennis. Badminton. Squash. Running. Track. Cross-country. American football (gridiron). Soccer. Rugby. Walking. Race walking.

Sports injury where stretch may be useful
Anterior compartment syndrome. Medial tibial pain syndrome (shin splints). Ankle sprain. Peroneal tendon subluxation. Peroneal tendonitis.

Additional information for performing this stretch correctly
If need be, hold onto something for balance.

Complementary stretch
109.

111: FRONT CROSS-OVER SHIN STRETCH

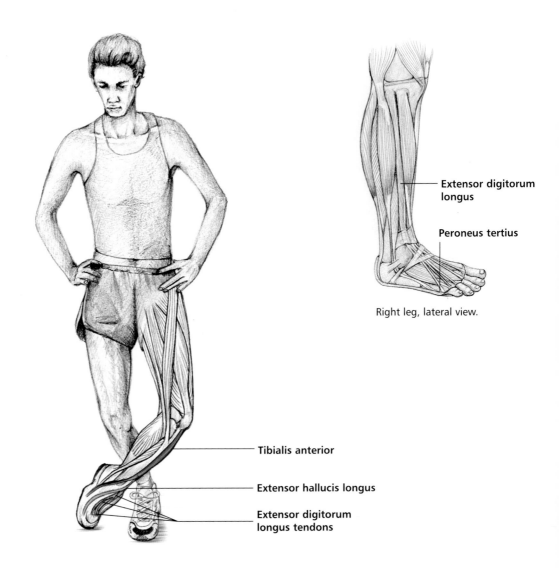

Extensor digitorum longus

Peroneus tertius

Right leg, lateral view.

Tibialis anterior

Extensor hallucis longus

Extensor digitorum longus tendons

Technique
Stand upright and place the top of your toes on the ground in front of your other foot. Slowly bend your other leg to force your ankle to the ground.

Muscles being stretched
Primary muscle: Tibialis anterior.
Secondary muscles: Extensor hallucis longus. Extensor digitorum longus. Peroneus tertius.

Sports that benefit from this stretch
Basketball. Netball. Boxing. Hiking. Backpacking. Mountaineering. Orienteering. Martial arts. Tennis. Badminton. Squash. Running. Track. Cross-country. American football (gridiron). Soccer. Rugby. Walking. Race walking.

Sports injury where stretch may be useful
Anterior compartment syndrome. Medial tibial pain syndrome (shin splints). Ankle sprain. Peroneal tendon subluxation. Peroneal tendonitis.

Additional information for performing this stretch correctly
Regulate the intensity of this stretch by lowering your body.

Complementary stretch
112.

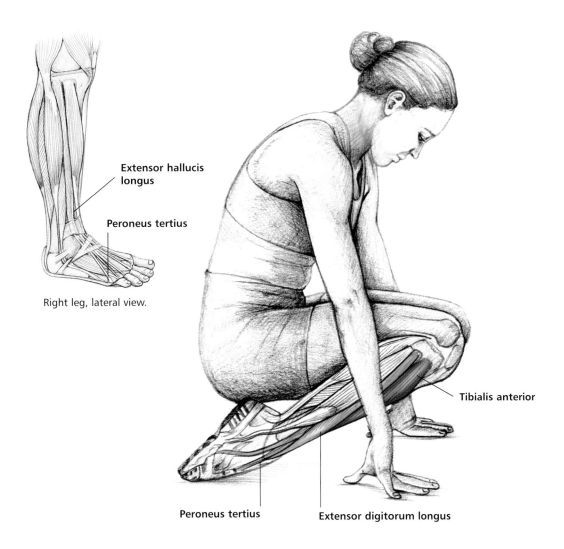

Extensor hallucis longus

Peroneus tertius

Right leg, lateral view.

Tibialis anterior

Peroneus tertius

Extensor digitorum longus

Technique

Sit with your knees and feet flat on the ground. Sit back on your ankles and keep your heels and knees together. Place your hands next to your knees and slowly lean backwards. Slowly raise your knees off the ground.

Muscles being stretched

Primary muscle: Tibialis anterior.
Secondary muscles: Extensor hallucis longus. Extensor digitorum longus. Peroneus tertius.

Sports that benefit from this stretch

Basketball. Netball. Boxing. Hiking. Backpacking. Mountaineering. Orienteering. Martial arts. Tennis. Badminton. Squash. Running. Track. Cross-country. American football (gridiron). Soccer. Rugby. Walking. Race walking.

Sports injury where stretch may be useful

Anterior compartment syndrome. Medial tibial pain syndrome (shin splints). Ankle sprain. Peroneal tendon subluxation. Peroneal tendonitis.

Common problems and additional information for performing this stretch correctly

This stretch can put a lot of pressure on your knees and ankles. Do not attempt this stretch if you suffer from knee or ankle pain.

Complementary stretch

110.

113: ANKLE ROTATION STRETCH

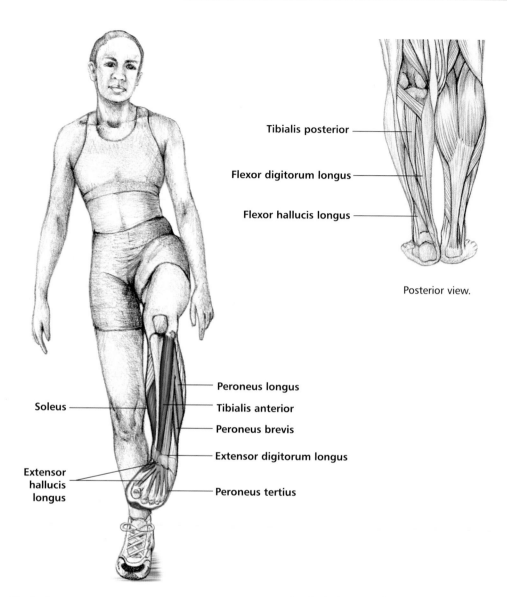

Tibialis posterior

Flexor digitorum longus

Flexor hallucis longus

Posterior view.

Soleus

Extensor hallucis longus

Peroneus longus

Tibialis anterior

Peroneus brevis

Extensor digitorum longus

Peroneus tertius

Technique
Raise one foot off the ground and slowly rotate your foot and ankle in all directions.

Muscles being stretched
Primary muscles: Soleus. Tibialis anterior. Secondary muscles: Extensor hallucis longus. Extensor digitorum longus. Peroneus longus, brevis and tertius. Tibialis posterior. Flexor hallucis longus. Flexor digitorum longus.

Sports that benefit from this stretch
Basketball. Netball. Boxing. Hiking. Backpacking. Mountaineering. Orienteering. Martial arts. Tennis. Badminton. Squash. Running. Track. Cross-country. American football (gridiron). Soccer. Rugby. Walking. Race walking.

Sports that benefit from this stretch
Anterior compartment syndrome. Medial tibial pain syndrome (shin splints). Ankle sprain. Posterior tibial tendonitis. Peroneal tendon subluxation. Peroneal tendonitis.

Additional information for performing this stretch correctly
If need be, hold onto something for balance.

Complementary stretches
111, 102.

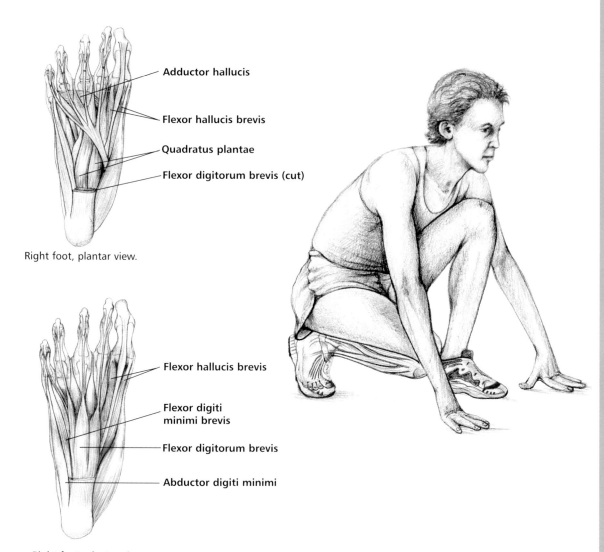

Right foot, plantar view.

- Adductor hallucis
- Flexor hallucis brevis
- Quadratus plantae
- Flexor digitorum brevis (cut)

Right foot, plantar view.

- Flexor hallucis brevis
- Flexor digiti minimi brevis
- Flexor digitorum brevis
- Abductor digiti minimi

Technique
Kneel on one foot with your hands on the ground. Place your body weight over your knee and slowly move your knee forward. Keep your toes on the ground and arch your foot.

Muscles being stretched
Primary muscles: Flexor digitorum brevis. Abductor hallucis. Abductor digiti minimi. Quadratus plantae.
Secondary muscles: Flexor hallucis brevis. Adductor hallucis. Flexor digiti minimi brevis.

Sports that benefit from this stretch
Basketball. Netball. Boxing. Cycling. Hiking. Backpacking. Mountaineering. Orienteering. Martial arts. Tennis. Badminton. Squash. Running. Track. Cross-country. American football (gridiron). Soccer. Rugby. Surfing. Walking. Race walking.

Sports injury where stretch may be useful
Posterior tibial tendonitis. Peroneal tendon subluxation. Peroneal tendonitis. Flexor tendonitis. Sesamoiditis. Plantar fasciitis.

Common problems and additional information for performing this stretch correctly
The muscles and tendons underneath the foot can be very tight; do not apply too much force too quickly when doing this stretch.

Complementary stretch
107.

Glossary of Medical Terms

Achilles tendonitis Inflammation of the Achilles tendon.

Adhesive capsulitis Adhesive inflammation between the joint capsule and the peripheral articular cartilage of the shoulder. Causes pain, stiffness, and limitation of movement. Also known as frozen shoulder.

Ankylosing spondylitis Form of degenerative joint disease that affects the spine. Systemic illness, producing pain and stiffness as a result of inflammation of the sacroiliac, intervertebral, and costovertebral joints.

Anterior tibial compartment syndrome Rapid swelling, increased tension, and pain of the anterior tibial compartment of the leg. Usually a history of excessive exertion.

Arthropathy Any joint disease.

Articular dysfunction Disturbance, impairment, or abnormality of a joint.

Avulsion fracture Indirect fracture caused by compressive forces from direct trauma or excessive tensile forces.

Bursa Fibrous sac membrane containing synovial fluid, typically found between tendons and bones. It acts to reduce friction during movement.

Bursitis Inflammation of the bursa, e.g. subdeltoid bursa.

Calcific tendonitis Inflammation and calcification of the subacromial or subdeltoid bursa. This results in pain, and limitation of movement of the shoulder.

Capsulitis Inflammation of a capsule, e.g. joint.

Carpal tunnel syndrome Compression of the median nerve as it passes through the carpal tunnel, leading to pain and tingling in the hand.

Cervical nerve stretch syndrome Condition caused by irritation or compression of the cervical nerve roots by a protruding disc.

Coccydynia Pain in the coccyx and neighbouring region. Also known as coccygodynia.

Compartment syndrome Condition in which increased intramuscular pressure impedes blood flow and function of tissues within that compartment.

Discogenic pain Pain caused by derangement of an intervertebral disc.

Dislocation The displacement of any part, especially of a bone.

Epicondylitis Inflammation and microrupturing of the soft tissues on the epicondyles of the distal humerus.

Fasciitis Inflammation of the fascia surrounding portions of a muscle.

Frozen shoulder syndrome see adhesive capsulitis.

Golfer's elbow Inflammation of the medial epicondyle of the humerus caused by activities (e.g. golf) that involve gripping and twisting, especially when there is a forceful grip.

Heel spur Bony spur from the calcaneum.

Iliotibial band syndrome Pain/ inflammation of the iliotibial band (ITB), a non-elastic collagen cord stretching from the pelvis to below the knee. There are various biomechanical causes.
Impingement syndrome Chronic condition caused by a repetitive overhead activity that damages the glenoid labrum, long head of the biceps brachii, and subacromial bursa.
Inflammation A localized protective response caused by injury to tissues. Characterized by pain, heat, redness, swelling, and loss of function.

Lordosis Excessive convex curve in the lumbar region of the spine.

Medial tibial pain syndrome Rapid swelling, increased tension, and pain of the medial tibial compartment of the leg. Usually a history of excessive exertion. Also known as shin splints.

Neuritis Inflammation of a nerve, with pain and tenderness.

Osteitis Inflammation of a bone, causing enlargement of the bone, tenderness, and a dull, aching pain.
Osteitis pubis A symptom-producing inflammatory condition of the pubic bones in the region of the symphysis. May be caused by a variety of conditions including degenerative changes.
Osteoarthritis Non-inflammatory degenerative joint disease, characterized by degeneration of the articular cartilage, hypertrophy of bone at the margins, and changes in the synovial membrane. Seen particularly in older persons.

Patellofemoral pain syndrome Excessive pain pertaining to the patella and femur.
Piriformis syndrome Condition resulting from the muscle being inflamed, shortened, or in spasm, causing impingement on the sciatic nerve. Causes pain and tingling in the posterior thigh and buttock. Occurs more frequently in women than men (ratio 6:1).

Repetitive strain injury (RSI) Refers to any overuse condition, such as strain, or tendonitis in any part of the body.
Rheumatoid arthritis Autoimmune disease, in which the immune system attacks the body's own tissues. Causes inflammation of many parts of the body.
Rotator cuff Helps hold the head of the humerus in contact with the glenoid cavity (fossa, socket) of the scapula during movements of the shoulder, thus helping to prevent dislocation of the joint. Comprises of: supraspinatus, infraspinatus, teres minor, and subscapularis.
Rupture Forcible tearing or disruption of tissue.

Sacroiliitis Inflammation (arthritis) in the sacroiliac joint.
Scapulocostal syndrome Pain in the superior or posterior aspect of the shoulder girdle, as a result of long-standing alteration of the relationship of the scapula and the posterior thoracic wall.
Scoliosis Lateral rotational spinal curvature.
Sesamoid bone Small nodular bones embedded in a tendon or joint.
Sesamoiditis Inflammation of the sesamoid bones and surrounding structures.
Shin splints see medial tibial pain syndrome /anterior tibial compartment syndrome.

Snapping hip syndrome Possibly caused by tight ligaments and tendons passing over bony prominences. Internal snapping mainly caused by the suction phenomenon, occurring during exercises such as sit-ups. External snapping usually as a result of the gluteus maximus clicking over the greater trochanter. Common in dancers and young athletes. Also known as clicking hip syndrome.

Sprain Joint injury in which some of the fibres of a supporting ligament are ruptured.

Strain An overstretching or overexertion of some part of the musculature.

Subluxation An incomplete or partial dislocation.

Tendonitis Inflammation of a tendon. Also known as tendinitis.

Tennis elbow Tendonitis of the muscles of the back of the forearm at their insertion. Caused by excessive hammering or sawing type movements, or a tense, awkward grip on a tennis racquet.

Tenosynovitis Inflammation of a tendon sheath.

Thrower's elbow Repetitive stress to the medial collateral ligament.

Torticollis Contracted state of the cervical muscles, producing twisting of the neck.

Trochanteric bursitis Trochanteric bursa lies between gluteus maximus and the posterolateral surface of the greater trochanter. Bursitis may occur if flexibility of the iliotibial band (ITB) is reduced.

Ulnar tunnel syndrome The ulnar nerve runs down the inside of the forearm to the heel of the hand. Excessive pressure on this nerve can cause numbness and tingling that is confined to the little finger and the outside of the ring finger. Usually not caused by repetitive motions.

Whiplash Nonspecific term applied to injury to the spine and spinal cord at C4/C5, occurring as the result of rapid acceleration/deceleration of the body.

Wry neck see torticollis.

Appendix

At-a-Glance Summary of Stretches for Sports / Sports Injuries

Sports	Stretches
American football (gridiron)	001–006; 028–031; 035–039; 041–114
Archery	002; 006–011; 032; 042–044
Athletics throwing field events	007–027
Athletics field events	042–044
Backpacking	012–017; 028–031; 035–039; 041–114
Badminton	007–027; 032; 035; 036; 041–044; 93–114
Baseball	007–031; 035; 036; 041–044; 048–050
Basketball	012–018; 022–031; 033; 034; 037–040; 044; 069–114
Boxing	001–011; 028–032; 036; 044; 048–050; 093–114
Canoeing	007–032; 035; 036; 041–044; 048–050; 057; 058
Cricket	007–031; 035; 036; 041–044; 048; 050
Cross-country	028–031; 037–039; 041–047; 051–114
Cycling	003–006; 032; 035–039; 041–047; 051–108
Field hockey	022–031; 035–039; 041–108
Golf	006–011; 028–032; 035; 036; 041–044
Hiking	012–017; 028–031; 035–039; 041–114
Ice hockey	022–031; 036–039; 041–108
Ice-skating	028–031; 037–039; 045–047; 051–108
Inline skating	028–031; 037–039; 045–047; 051–071; 082–108
Kayaking	007–032; 035; 036; 041–044; 048–050; 057; 058
Martial arts	019–031; 037–039; 045–114
Mountaineering	012–017; 028–031; 035–039; 041–114
Netball	012–018; 022–031; 033; 034; 037–040; 044; 069–114
Orienteering	012–017; 028–031; 035–039; 041–114
Race walking	028–031; 036–039; 041–047; 051–114
Roller-skating	028–031; 037–039; 045–047; 051–108
Rowing	007–032; 035; 036; 041–044; 048–050; 057; 058
Rugby	001–006; 028; 030; 031; 035–039; 041–114
Running	028–031; 036–039; 041–047; 051–114
Snow skiing	028–032; 037–039; 045–047; 051–108
Soccer	028–031; 037–039; 041–047; 051–114
Softball	007–011; 022–031; 035; 036; 041–044; 048–050
Squash	007–027; 032; 035; 036; 041–044; 093–114
Surfing	028–031; 037–039; 045; 046; 048–050; 064–108
Swimming	001–027; 032–036; 040–044; 093–108
Tennis	007–027; 032; 035; 036; 041–044; 093–114
Track	028–031; 037–039; 041–047; 051–114
Volleyball	018; 022–027; 033; 034; 040
Walking	028–031; 036–039; 041–046; 051–114
Water skiing	028–032; 037–039; 045–047; 051–108
Wrestling	001–006; 019–031; 045–050; 069–092

Sports Injuries

Stretches

Sports Injuries	Stretches
Abdominal muscle strain	028–031; 042–044; 047–050
Achilles tendonitis	079; 080; 097–108
Achilles tendon strain	079; 080; 097–108
Acromioclavicular separation	007–011; 013–017; 019–021
Adhesive capsulitis	007–017; 019–021
Ankle sprain	109–113
Anterior compartment syndrome	109–113
Avulsion fracture in the pelvic area	064–068; 082–088
Back ligament sprain	033; 035; 036; 041–044
Lower	037–040; 045–051; 059; 061; 069–078; 081
Upper	032; 034
Back muscle strain	033; 035; 036; 041–044
Lower	037–040; 045–051; 059; 061; 069–078; 081
Upper	032; 034
Bicepital tendonitis	011; 013; 014; 022
Biceps strain	011; 013; 014; 022
Biceps tendon rupture	011; 013; 014; 022
Calf strain	071–074; 076–078; 081; 097–108
Carpel tunnel syndrome	023–027
Cervical nerve stretch syndrome	001–006; 032; 034–036; 041
Chest strain	011–017; 031
Dislocation	007–011; 013–017; 019–021
Elbow bursitis	018; 022
Elbow dislocation	018; 022
Elbow sprain	018
Elbow strain	022
Flexor tendonitis	114
Frozen shoulder, *see* adhesive capsulitis	
Golfer's elbow	022–027
Groin strain	055–058; 082–088
Hamstring strain	037–039; 059; 061; 069–081; 087; 088; 098; 099
Hip flexor strain	029; 030; 064–067
Iliopsoas tendonitis	029; 030; 064–068
Iliotibial band syndrome	045–047; 051; 059; 061; 089–092
Impingement syndrome	007–017; 019–021
Medial tibial pain syndrome	079; 080; 097–113
Neck muscle strain	001–006; 032; 034–036; 041
Neck sprain, *see* whiplash	

Sports Injuries	Stretches
Osteitis pubis	064–068; 082–088
Patellar tendonitis	065–068
Patellofemoral pain syndrome	065–068
Pectoral muscle insertion inflammation	011–017; 031
Peroneal tendonitis	109–114
Peroneal tendon subluxation	109–114
Piriformis syndrome	052–058; 060; 062; 063; 082–088
Plantar fasciitis	114
Posterior tibial tendonitis	101–108; 113; 114
Quadriceps strain	064–068
Quadriceps tendonitis	064–068
Rotator cuff tendonitis	007–017; 019–021
Sesamoiditis	114
Shin splints, *see* medial tibial pain syndrome	
Shoulder bursitis	007–017; 019–021
Snapping hip syndrome	052–058; 060; 062; 063
Sternoclavicular separation	007–011; 013–017; 019–021
Subluxation	007–011; 013–017; 019–021
Subluxing kneecap	065–068
Tendonitis of the adductor muscles	055–058; 082–088
Tennis elbow	022–027
Thrower's elbow	022–027
Torticollis, *see* wryneck	
Triceps tendon rupture	018
Trochanteric bursitis	052–058; 060; 062–068; 082–092
Ulnar tunnel syndrome	023–027
Whiplash	001–006; 032; 034–036; 041
Wrist dislocation	023–027
Wrist sprain	023–027
Wrist tendonitis	023–027
Wryneck	001–006; 032; 034–036; 041

Resources

Alter, M.J.: 1998. *Sports Stretch.* Human Kinetics. IL, USA

Anderson, D.M. (chief lexicographer): 2003. *Dorland's Illustrated Medical Dictionary, 30th edition.* Saunders, an imprint of Elsevier. Philadelphia, USA

Anderson, R.A.: 1981. *Stretching.* Shelter Publications. CA, USA

Appleton, B.D.: 1998. *Stretching and Flexibility.* Self-published

Arnheim, D.D.: 1989. *Modern Principles of Athletic Training.* Times Mirror. MO, USA

Delavier, F.: 2006. *Strength Training Anatomy, 2e.* Human Kinetics. IL, USA

Goldspink, G.: 1968. Sarcomere Length During Post-natal Growth and Mammalian Muscle Fibers. *J. of Cell Science,* **3**(4) : 539-548

Gummerson, T.: 1990. *Mobility Training for the Martial Arts.* A & C Black. London, UK

Jarmey, C.: 2003. *The Concise Book of Muscles.* Lotus Publishing/ North Atlantic Books. Chichester, UK/ Berkeley, USA

Kurz, T.: 2003. *Stretching Scientifically.* Stadion Publishing Company. VT, USA

Lamb, D.R.: 1984. *Physiology of Exercise.* Macmillan Publishing Co. NY, USA

Laughlin, K.: 1999. *Stretching and Flexibility.* Simon & Schuster. NSW, Australia

Sang, K.H.: 2004. *Ultimate Flexibility.* Turtle Press. CT, USA

Tortora, G.J. & Anagnostakos, N.P.: 1990. *Principles of Anatomy and Physiology.* Harper & Row. NY, USA

Walker, B.E.: 1998. *The Stretching Handbook.* Walkerbout Health. Qld, Australia

Williams, P.E., & Goldspink, G.: 1971. Longitudinal Growth of Striated Muscle Fibers. *J. of Cell Science,* **9**(3): 751-767

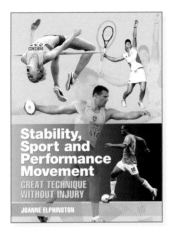

Stability, Sport, and Performance Movement

Joanne Elphinston

978 1 905367 09 2 (UK)/978 1 55643 746 5 (US); **£24.99/$32.95**; 352 pages; 265 mm x 194 mm; 320 colour illustrations; paperback

In every sport, there are athletes who represent true technical excellence. Their movement seems effortless, controlled and efficient: they create and control forces in the most effective way.

The building blocks of stability, mobility, symmetry, and balance provide the foundation for sports movement development and injury resistance. These elements combine to prevent the physical restrictions, imbalances and inefficient muscle recruitment patterns which can block athletes from meeting their movement goals. The right muscles firing at the right time and in the right sequence can enable athletes to achieve their full physical potential.

Full of colour photographs and images to illustrate the techniques and theories involved, *Stability, Sport, and Performance Movement* introduces functional stability principles as they apply to sporting movement. A comprehensive chapter on movement testing is followed with four chapters of integrated exercise techniques, which clearly demonstrate form and progression from early activation through to high-level neuromuscular drills. Programmes and clinical examples help the reader to appreciate the application of this approach across a variety of sports.

It is an approach that has been used with international-level athletes in disciplines as diverse as swimming, badminton, gymnastics, karate, cycling, weight lifting, basketball, athletics, snow sports, football, golf, equestrian sports, and tennis. However, it is applicable and relevant across all age groups and ability levels, from beginners through to veterans. Effective adult movement starts with great foundations, so a dedicated chapter on establishing stable controlled movement in children is included.

Joanne Elphinston, is a Performance Consultant, international lecturer and physiotherapist working with elite and professional athletes including Olympic, Commonwealth and World Championship medallists, Premiership footballers and professional golfers. Joanne is a consultant on Performance Movement to the British Olympic Association, as well as advising professional sporting organisations on technical movement enhancement for performance, injury prevention and rehabilitation. She also has extensive experience in child and adolescent movement development for sport and its progression into senior competition.

Gloss Laminated Wall Charts

Using drawings taken from the best-selling *The Anatomy of Stretching*, these beautifully illustrated wall charts show exactly what is happening during a stretch. Each of the 16 key stretches illustrates the primary and secondary muscles worked, showing how to perform each stretch and highlight sports injuries for which each stretch will be beneficial.

Aimed at fitness professionals, physical therapists, sports scientists, or anyone involved in sport, these charts will help explain what is happening during a stretch, how the stretch can assist in recovery from injury, and add colour to any gym or treatment room wall.

PRICE: **£10.99** plus VAT
FORMAT: 995mm x 740mm

Upper Body Stretches
(ISBN 978 1 905367 14 6)

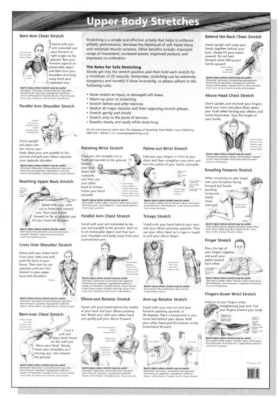

Lower Body Stretches
(ISBN 978 1 905367 15 3)

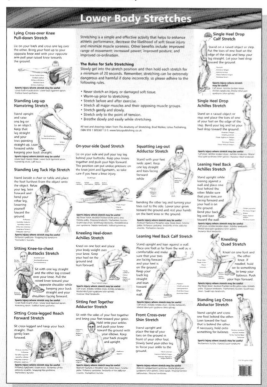

Neck, Back and Core Stretches
(ISBN 978 1 905367 16 0)

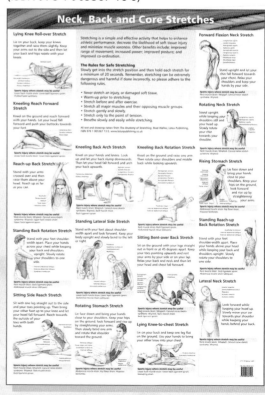